CELL BIOLOGY RESEARCH PROGRESS

GANGLION CELLS

MORPHOLOGY, FUNCTIONAL DEVELOPMENT AND ROLE IN DISEASE

CELL BIOLOGY RESEARCH PROGRESS

Additional books in this series can be found on Nova's website under the Series tab.

Additional e-books in this series can be found on Nova's website under the e-book tab.

CELL BIOLOGY RESEARCH PROGRESS

GANGLION CELLS

MORPHOLOGY, FUNCTIONAL DEVELOPMENT AND ROLE IN DISEASE

LIORA G. VLASTIMIL
EDITOR

New York

For permission to use material from this book please contact us:
Telephone 631-231-7269; Fax 631-231-8175
Web Site: http://www.novapublishers.com

Library of Congress Cataloging-in-Publication Data

ISBN: 978-1-63117-432-2

Library of Congress Control Number: 2014932934

Published by Nova Science Publishers, Inc. † New York

CONTENTS

PREFACE

The ability to observe the world around us through sight provides us with many advantages we may take for granted daily. We are able to recognize a hazard well in advance because we see it; we can find allies because we see them. Further, thanks to the perception of the world that gives us sight, we can collect information to help us develop feelings, such as trust in others, love and sensations, like beauty. However, the mechanism to enjoy this capability is really complex, starting with the structure responsible for receiving, processing and transmitting information to the brain. This book discusses the ways in which ganglion cells are used in the nervous system, as well as its morphology, functional development and role in diseases.

Chapter 1 - The orderly, retinotopic mapping of retinal ganglion cell (RGC) axon terminals within the visual centers of the brain is critical to functional visual perception. More than 50 years ago, Roger Sperry developed the chemoaffinity model to explain the intrinsic ability of regenerating RGC axons to find and synapse in the appropriate retinotopic organization within the optic tectum in the goldfish, *Carassius auratus*. He proposed that orthogonal gradients of signaling molecules could function as Cartesian coordinate systems within the retina and brain to specify physical addresses of RGCs and their post-syanptic targets. These chemoaffinity molecules, subsequently identified as ephrins (EFN) and tyrosine kinase ephrin receptors (EPH), have been shown to play a vital role in establishing topographic maps of connectivity throughout the visual and other sensory systems within the central nervous system. This chapter presents a comprehensive review of the discovery, structure, signal transduction, expression patterns and transcriptional regulation of EPH receptors, ephrin ligands and EPH/EFN signaling in RGCs during visual system development and in diseases affecting the optic nerve.

Chapter 2 - Mammalian photoreception requires the presence of photosensitive cells in the retina. This process takes place thanks to a protein (opsin), which contains a cromophore. Rods and cones allow mammals, and other multiple species, to see the world around them. Rods and cones were thought to be the only photoreceptors until the last decades. The discovery of a new opsin (melanopsin) inside other retinal cells has finished with the traditional exclusivity of rods and cones as photosensitive cells. In mammals, these cells are localized in the Ganglion Cell Layer. There is a ganglion cell type that contains this photopigment, the melanopsin ganglion cells, commonly known as ipRGCs (intrinsically photosensitive retinal ganglion cells). These cells appear to have a key role in regulating certain aspects of the visual system not related to image formation, as well as various physiological functions fundamental for the organism: Melanopsin is an important regulator of the circadian clock.

Earlier studies showed how blind individuals with degenerated rod and cone photoreceptors still maintained photoentrainment and the pupillary light reflex. The presence of another photoreceptor was obvious. Melanopsin-containing cells were found in mouse and human retinal ganglion cells, but other animals had amacrine and horizontal cells that also expressed melanopsin. Melanopsin ganglion cells were regarded as the new type of photoreceptor. However, recent studies indicate that ipRGCs are composed of different subtypes. The relation between subtype and function is not always clear. Some of these subtypes share targets in the central nervous system (or even share physiological functions), but they have important morphological differences.

Nowadays, the scientific community accepts the role of the different ipRGCs in non-visual processes, whereas rods and cones are involved in image formation. It is very interesting to study the differences between melanopsin retinal ganglion cells and classical photoreceptors, since their physiological functions are not the only differences. In addition, their molecular requirements and their photochemical properties show a different evolutionary origin. Understanding the evolution and functions of visual and non-visual systems is crucial to understand the functional differences among opsins.

Chapter 3 - The DBA/2J mouse is a common animal model of glaucoma. The intraocular pressure increases with age, and retinal ganglion cells (RGC) degenerate, usually starting at an age of approximately six months. In this chapter, the authors show how RGC degeneration in two-year-old DBA/2J mice has almost reached an end-point. The authors investigated visual function in these animals using electroretinography (ERG) and visual evoked potentials (VEP), and the authors checked the number of remaining RGC by retrograde staining. Almost no RGC were left in the retina, and VEP were hardly recordable. Surprisingly, also ERG amplitudes of scotopic a-waves and b-waves, photopic b-waves and oscillatory potentials were decreased significantly by approximately 40% compared to amplitudes measured in age-matched C57BL/6J mice. The latencies were not changed in DBA/2J mice compared to controls, and so were the ratios between amplitudes of a-waves, b-waves and oscillatory potentials. The author's results indicate that, in addition to degeneration of RGC, also photoreceptors are affected by pathological processes in the eye caused by the mutations present in DBA/2J mice.

Chapter 4 - Dorsal root ganglion (DRG) neurons are constituents of the peripheral sensory nervous system, and methods for their primary culture from embryonic, neonatal, and adult animals have been established. Because some biological properties of DRG neurons can change with maturation and aging, adult DRG neurons appear to be a better choice for studies on axonal regeneration after injury and peripheral neuropathies than immature neurons. In dissociated cell culture, each of the ganglion neurons is mechanically and enzymatically isolated and seeded in a substrate-coated culture dish. Because of the good yield of ganglion neurons with high purity and viability, various assays can be performed on these neurons (e.g., cell attachment, cell viability, neurite outgrowth activity, electrophysiology, and immunocytochemistry). In explant culture, ganglia associated with nerve fibers are embedded in a collagen gel or Matrigel, and the number and length of neurites outgrowing from nerve-transected terminals are measured. Because cell–cell interactions are maintained in an explanted tissue, it is likely that an explant culture system mimics nerve regeneration *in vivo* better than a dissociated cell culture system. Using these culture systems, the authors investigated mechanisms of action of several different molecules that regulate axonal regeneration (e.g., ciliary neurotrophic factor, galectin-1, exendin-4, and chondroitin sulfate proteoglycans). In addition, these culture methods have been applied to animal models of aging and diseases (e.g., diabetes, G_{M2} gangliosidosis, and systemic lupus erythematosus) to elucidate the pathogenesis of neurological disorders that result from those conditions.

In: Ganglion Cells
Editor: Liora G. Vlastimil

ISBN: 978-1-63117-432-2

Chapter 1

EPH-EPHRIN SIGNALING IN RETINAL GANGLION CELLS

Deborah C. Otteson[1,*] ***and Tihomira D. Petkova***
College of Optometry, University of Houston, Houston, TX, US

ABSTRACT

The orderly, retinotopic mapping of retinal ganglion cell (RGC) axon terminals within the visual centers of the brain is critical to functional visual perception. More than 50 years ago, Roger Sperry developed the chemoaffinity model to explain the intrinsic ability of regenerating RGC axons to find and synapse in the appropriate retinotopic organization within the optic tectum in the goldfish, *Carassius auratus*. He proposed that orthogonal gradients of signaling molecules could function as Cartesian coordinate systems within the retina and brain to specify physical addresses of RGCs and their post-syanptic targets. These chemoaffinity molecules, subsequently identified as ephrins (EFN) and tyrosine kinase ephrin receptors (EPH), have been shown to play a vital role in establishing topographic maps of connectivity throughout the visual and other sensory systems within the central nervous system. This chapter presents a comprehensive review of the discovery, structure, signal transduction, expression patterns and transcriptional regulation of EPH receptors, ephrin ligands and EPH/EFN signaling in RGCs during visual system development and in diseases affecting the optic nerve.

---

* Corresponding author. E-mail: dotteson@optometry.uh.edu; Phone: 713-743-1952.

1. Introduction

A fundamental problem facing developing neurons is how to locate and connect with the appropriate post-synaptic cells. This is most clearly problematic for projection neurons, including retinal ganglion cells (RGCs), which must extend their axons significant distances to reach their post-synaptic targets. For optic nerve development, the problem of connectivity can be subdivided into a series of tasks or decision points. Upon withdrawal from the cell cycle, RGCs must first project their axons towards the nascent optic disc. After entering the ventral optic stalk, axons extend to the ventral diencephalon where they must either decussate or remain ipsilateral before entering the optic tract. Upon exiting the optic tract, the axons then must find and synapse with the appropriate target cells in the visual centers of the brain.

Superimposed on the basic problems of axon guidance is the establishment of the fundamental retinotopic organization of the visual system. This organization is such that the relative positions of RGC cell bodies within the retina are maintained in the location of their synaptic terminals within each of the visual centers in the brain. Retinotopic organization is maintained at all levels of the visual system, from the direct synaptic targets of RGC axons (e.g., superior colliculus/optic tectum and lateral geniculate nucleus) to the visual cortex (V1 and beyond), where the mapping becomes increasingly complex. Topographic mapping is a key characteristic of all sensory and motor systems and is most commonly represented in classical neuroanatomy as the homunculus of the sensory and motor cortices. Forward and reverse signaling through ephrin receptors (EPH) and ephrin ligands (EFN) is a major mechanism specifying the positional information that underlies the formation of topographic maps throughout the central nervous systems.

In the visual projections, two major roles for EPH/ephrin signaling are (1) to mediate appropriate decussation of the ipsilateral and contralateral components of the optic nerve at the optic chiasm, and (2) to provide positional information that establishes the initial patterns of connectivity. Initial maps are subsequently refined, in part, through activity-dependent mechanisms to generate the final retinotopic maps [1]. This chapter examines the discovery, structure, signal transduction, expression patterns and transcriptional regulation of EPH receptors, ephrin ligands and EPH/EFN signaling in RGCs during visual system development and in diseases affecting the optic nerve.

Throughout this chapter, the emphasis will be on data from several vertebrate species (fish, chick and mouse) with primarily crossed visual pathways and major projections to the optic tectum/superior colliculus. This will be supplemented with key findings from ferret, human and primates, which have increased binocular vision with a greater ipsilateral component to the visual system and significant projections to the lateral geniculate nucleus.

Note: We have observed the following convention when using gene name abbreviations: for a gene or mRNA, all letters will be in italics. For human genes/mRNA, all letters will be capitalized (*EPHA5*), for mouse or rat genes the first letter will be capitalized (*EphA5*) and for chick, fish or other non-mammalian vertebrates, first letter is lower case (*ephA5*). For proteins, all capital letters without italics will be used for all species (EPHA5) [2, 3].

2. Chemoaffinity and Retinotectal Mapping

It has been 50 years since Sperry first proposed that the orderly connectivity of retinal ganglion cell axons in the brain could be regulated by chemotactic signals [4]. In studies of optic nerve regeneration in goldfish, Sperry and colleagues demonstrated that regenerating retinal ganglion cell axons did not connect randomly to post synaptic cells in the optic tectum, nor did they connect with the first post synaptic cell they encountered. Instead, RGC axons bypassed inappropriate targets to synapse in the topographically appropriate location. This provided the foundation for Sperry's chemoaffinity theory that orthogonal gradients of chemotactic molecules in the retina and in the optic tectum provide the positional information that specify where axons will terminate. "These separate gradients successively superimposed on the retinal and tectal fields and surroundings would stamp each cell with its appropriate latitude and longitude expressed in a kind of chemical code with matching values between the retinal and tectal maps" [4].

By 1970, the chemoaffinity theory had begun to garner criticism, in part because the proposed chemoaffinity molecules had not been identified. Furthermore, strict chemoaffinity labels appeared to be insufficient to explain observed plasticity within the visual system. There were also questions regarding the feasibility of having precise chemical signatures for every cell that could specify one-to-one matching of an RGC to its ideal post-synaptic cell. It was increasingly clear that the number of proteins in the retina was insufficient to generate a unique chemical signature for each RGC. More importantly, partial ablation of the optic tectum prior to innervation did not disrupt the overall topographic organization of RGC axon terminals but led to a compression of the maps into the remaining available space [5]. This led Gaze and Keating to state: "It must be acknowledged that there is, in fact, no evidence that requires the view that the formation of synapses at specific sites is due to any form of neuronal chemospecificity" [6].

However, the evidence for orderly patterns of connectivity between the retina and brain was compelling and the controversy over mechanisms stimulated continued research in this field. With development of new technologies, such as cell culture and monoclonal antibody production, there were increasing efforts to identify molecules that were expressed in spatially restricted patterns within the retina and tectum that could serve as chemoaffinity labels. In co-cultures, retinal ganglion cells from the ventral hemiretina preferentially adhered to anterior halves of the optic tectum, whereas dorsal retinal cells preferred posterior tectal halves [7]. Importantly, trypsinization of the retinal cells temporarily eliminated the preferential adhesion, demonstrating that cell surface proteins were responsible for the spatial specificities of retinal/tectal cell adhesion. Consistent with the presence of topographically distributed cell surface molecules, dissociated cells from chick retina showed a dorsal/ventral gradient of homotypic cell adhesion preferences, with dorsal retinal cells binding with higher affinity to dorsal cells and ventral binding preferentially to ventral cells [8]. Using monoclonal antibodies, the TOP (toponymic) antigen was found to be differentially expressed across the retina, with highest expression in the dorso-posterior portion of the retina [9]. Other molecules expressed in graded patterns were subsequently discovered, including 9-O-acetyl GD3 [10] and TRAP (temporal retinal axon protein) [11] in the retina and RGM (repulsive guidance molecule) in the optic tectum [12]. However, better functional data was needed to determine which, if any, of these were the elusive chemoaffinity molecules.

A key breakthrough came when Bonhoeffer developed an *in vitro* assay for ganglion cell axon outgrowth. In this system, retinal explants were given a choice to extend on monolayers of cells isolated from different portions of the optic tectum [13]. These experiments showed that in embryonic chick retina, temporal RGC axons avoided cells isolated from posterior tectum and showed a clear preference to extend on cells from the anterior tectum. However, the axons from nasal retina showed no obvious preference. Subsequent refinement of this assay to generate alternating stripes of tectal cell membranes made the "Stripe Assay" the mainstay of research to identify spatial and developmental differences in axon/substrate interactions and led to the identification and validation of candidate molecules for the elusive chemoaffinity signals [14]. Among the molecules identified, the ephrin receptor tyrosine kinases (EPH) and ephrin ligands (EFN) emerged as key players in retinotopic mapping of the retinocollicular and retinogeniculate pathways, as well as in connectivity and topographic mapping throughout the central nervous system.

3. EPH Receptors and Ephrin Ligands

3.1. History and Taxonomy

The first *EPH* receptor gene was cloned from erythropoietin-producing human hepato-cellular carcinoma cell line (ETL-1) and was a novel receptor tyrosine kinase that was structurally distinct from other known classes of receptor tyrosine kinses (e.g., epidermal growth factor receptors, insulin and insulin-related receptors, neurotrophin receptors, etc.) [15]. Currently, EPH receptors constitute the largest subfamily of receptor tyrosine kinase genes in vertebrates, consisting of 15 family members in total, with 13 of these present in mammals (Table 1). They are evolutionarily conserved, with orthologs identified in both invertebrates (e.g., sponges, nematodes, flies) and vertebrates (e.g., birds, amphibians, fish and mammals, including humans) [16-18]. Activation of signal transduction following receptor/ligand binding contributes to a wide variety of cellular processes, including cell-cell adhesion, vascular development, cancer *metastasis and* axon guidance, connectivity and synaptogenesis [19-24]

EPH receptors are divided into two subgroups, EPHA and EPHB, based on sequence and binding affinities to the ephrinA and ephrinB ligands [25]. Both EPHA and EPHB receptors are single pass tyrosine kinase receptors that range in size from 974-1038 amino acids in length in humans. Structurally, EPH receptors consist of an N-teminal, extracellular domain containing a single ligand binding domain, a cysteine rich domain and two fibronectin III domains, followed by a single transmembrane domain leading to the intracellular portion that contains a kinase domain, a SAM (sterile alpha motif) domain and a PDZ-binding domain the C-terminus (Figure 1) [26-28].

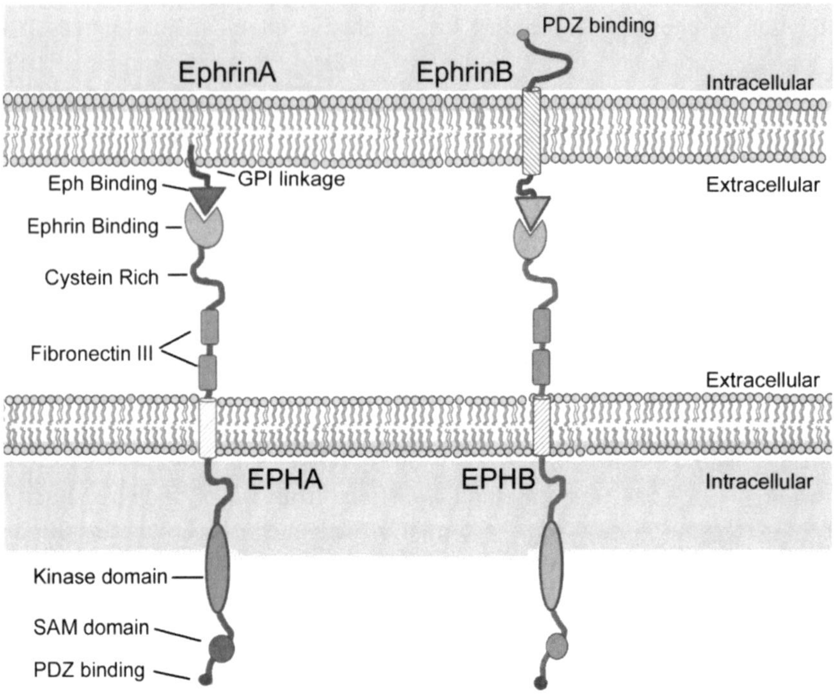

Figure 1. Structure of Eph/ephrin molecules.
Diagram showing interactions between ephrin expressing cell (top) and EPH receptor expressing cells showing structural domains of A-class (left) and B-class (right) ephrin receptors and ligands. SAM, sterile alpha motif; GPI, glycosyl-phosphatidylinositol. (adapted from Pasquale, 2010 [47]).

Ephrins (EFN) are the ligands for EPH receptors and are likewise divided into two groups, based on structural differences and their relative binding affinities for either EPHA or EPHB receptors (Figure 1). As with the EPH receptors, EFN ligands are found in both invertebrates and vertebrates and share structural and sequence homology across phylogenies [17, 29]. The five ephrinA ligands (EFNA1-A5) are small proteins (201-238 amino acids in human) consisting of an extracellular receptor binding domain anchored to the plasma membrane by a glycosyl-phosphatidylinositol (GPI) linkage [30]. The three ephrinB ligands (EFNB1-B3) are somewhat larger (333-346 amino acids in humans) and also contain an extracellular receptor binding domain. However, the ephrinB ligands are integral membrane proteins with both a hydrophobic transmembrane domain and a C-terminal cytoplasmic domain, which contains phosphorylation sites and a PDZ binding domain [31].

3.2. Ligand Binding

EPHA and EPHB receptors preferentially bind their corresponding class of ephrinA or ephrinB ligands to activate signal transduction cascades [32]. The ligand binding domain of the EPH receptors is localized in the extracellular, N-terminal globular domain [33, 34]. The adjacent cysteine rich domain may also contribute to binding, possibly through stabilization of the receptor/ligand interaction, however the fibronectin domains are not required for ligand binding, but instead contribute to receptor-receptor interactions associated with receptor clustering [35].

There is binding promiscuity within subclasses (EPHA/ephrinA or EPHB/ephrinB), with some receptors binding multiple ligands. Binding affinity for preferred ligands, in terms of their dissociation constants (K_D) are typically in the nanomolar range [36, 37]. In chick, ephrinA6 and ephrinA5 bind with high affinity (nM K_D) to EPHA3, EPHA4, EPHA5, EPHA7 and EPHA8, but with lower affinity (μM K_D) to EPHA6 [38]. There is, however, minimal cross talk between ligands and receptors of the opposite groups with two notable exceptions. EPHA4 can bind ephrinAs, as well as ephrinB2 and ephrinB3; EPHB2 can bind multiple ephrinBs, as well as ephrinA5. EPHA4 binds ephrinB2 and ephinB3 with estimated dissociation constants (K_D) in the nanomolar to micromolar range [39, 40]. This is lower than EPHA4's binding affinity for its preferred ligands (EFNA4, EFNA5: K_D in low nanomolar range), but similar to its binding affinity to non-preferred A-type ligands (EFNA1 and EFNA2: K_D in micromolar range) [37]. EPHB2 binds ephrinA5 with lower affinity than ephrinB1 or ephrinB2, but with higher affinity than to the other A type ephrins [41, 42-44].

EPHA4/ephrinB2 binding requires residues within the receptor's extracellular domain that are not required for binding of ephrinA ligands [39] and results in distinct changes in receptor conformation that results in receptor/ligand dimers that more closely resemble EPHB/ephrinB, rather than typical EPHA/ephrinA, complexes [45]. Based on X-ray crystallography, the EPHB2/ephrinA5 complexes also form heterodimers that are structurally distinct from the EPHB2/ephrinB2 heterodimers [41]. Whereas EPHB/ephrinB heterodimers cluster via receptor-receptor interaction, EPHB2/ephrinA5 clustering appears to rely more on the clustering of the ligands, independent of receptor/receptor interactions, to bring the ligand/receptor complexes into proximity for subsequent phosphorylation and activation of signal transduction.

4. EPH/Ephrin Intracellular Signaling

Following ligand binding, the basic steps of EPH/ephrin signaling include receptor/ligand clustering, internalization and initiation of signal transduction cascades. One unique feature of EPH receptors is that, unlike other tyrosine receptors, they bind to membrane bound ligands rather than secreted proteins. As a result, EPH receptor/ephrin binding can stimulate both "forward" signaling in the receptor-expressing cell and "reverse" signaling in the ligand-expressing cell [46, 47]. EPH/ephrin forward and reverse signaling involves a *trans* interaction between two cells and activation of signal transduction within the EPH and ephrin expressing cells [46, 48, 49]. There can also be *cis* interactions between EPH receptors and ligands expressed on the same cell, which appear to inhibit EPH/ephrin signaling [50-52]. The outcome and cellular response is influenced by the combinations and levels of the different receptors and ligands expressed by a cell and its neighbors, whether the clustered complexes are internalized by the receptor or the ligand bearing cell, and the other receptors or downstream effectors that may be associated with the receptor/ligand complexes.

4.1. Receptor/Ligand Clustering

To activate signal transduction, ephrin ligands and receptors must be clustered [53]. *In vivo*, ephrin ligands, most particularly the GPI-linked ephrinAs, tend to be pre-clustered in lipid rafts that can facilitate receptor recruitment and clustering [54-56]. Lipid rafts are microdomains within the plasma membrane which have been proposed to segregate components of different signaling pathways. For example, SRC-family kinases are known to be localized within lipid rafts [57, 58]. It has been proposed that ephrinAs and ephrinBs segregate into distinct membrane domains based on their distinct modes of membrane attachment (GPI-linked vs transmembrane) [59].

In vivo, ligand binding results in dimerization of EPH receptors via their intracellular SAM (sterile alpha motif) domains and leads to receptor clustering [27, 28]. *In vitro,* clustering of ephrins to activate EPH forward signaling is typically accomplished by conjugating the ephrins to Fc-immunoglobulins. Likewise, Fc-conjugated EPH receptors are used to bind to and stimulate reverse signaling through ephrin ligands. Unexpectedly, receptor clustering does not specifically require ligand binding or kinase activity, as EPHA3 receptors containing mutated ligand binding domains or lacking their cytoplasmic domains can be recruited into receptor clusters along with the native receptors [60].

Ligand clustering appears to influence EphB/ephrinB triggered growth cone collapse in retinal ganglion cells. In embryonic *Xenopus* retinal explants, pre-clustering of ephrinB1-Fc using antibodies against the Fc epitope induced a rapid and transient growth cone collapse, whereas without pre-clustering the ephrinB1-Fc had no effect [61]. These results suggested that activation of forward signaling through EPHB receptors required multimeric clustering, similar to what might be present in a lipid raft *in vivo*. In the same study, EPHB2-Fc induced a slow growth cone collapse, whereas pre-clustered EPHB2-Fc did not. Interestingly, the EPHB2-Fc induced growth cone collapse was dependent on endocytosis by the ligand expressing cells. It remains to be determined precisely why the pre-clustered EPHB2-Fc failed to elicit a cellular response, as both Fc- and pre-clustered Fc-conjugated receptors should be able to interact with the rafts of ephrin ligands resulting in subsequent multimerization.

4.2. EPH/Ephrin Forward Signaling

Activation of the signal transduction cascade downstream of EPH receptors activation and clustering begins with autophosphorylation of tyrosines in the juxtamembrane domain [27, 28, 33]. Once phosphorylated, EPH receptors interact with Sarc-homology (SH2) domain containing proteins (e.g., SRC, RasGAP, CRK and FYN) [26, 62, 63]. Both EPHA and EPHB forward signaling regulates a variety of guanine nucleotide exchange factors (GEFs), which, in turn, regulate the activity of members of the *Ras* family of small GTPases: RAC1, CDC42 and RHOA [64]. *Activation of tyrosine kinase activity of EPHB2 following ligand binding inactivates the RAS-MAPK pathway through p120RasGAP, resulting in reorganization of the actin cytoskeleton leading cell repulsion and growth cone collapse* [65]. Inhibition of cell migration and growth cone collapse can also result from direct RAS inhibition following phosphorylation of the RAS-effector binding domain by EPH receptors' tyrosine kinase activity [66]. For example, in chick retinal explant cultures, activation of EPHA forward signaling by soluble ephrinA5-Fc results in growth cone collapse of temporal RGCs that can be inhibited by overexpression of a constitutively active R-RAS [66]. Likewise, activation of EPHB3 reduces cell adhesion through phosphorylation of R-RAS at tyrosine

66, leading to down-regulation of integrin-mediated cell substrate binding [67].

A major mediator of EPHA forward signaling is ephexin, a guanine nucleotide exchange factor [68]. Ephexin is most highly expressed in the central nervous system, including the retina, where expression is detected in retinal ganglion cells and the inner nuclear layer of the rat retina, specifically during the developmental times associated with RGC connectivity [69]. Ephexin1 binds to the EPHA4 kinase domain and mediates the effects of ephrin signaling on cell motility and growth cone extension/collapse through phosphorylation of RHO family GTPases [69, 70]. Although in the absence of ephrinA, ephexin1 binding to EPHA signals for axon outgrowth, after activation of EPHA4 by ephrinA1 binding, ephexin1 preferentially activates RHOA GTPase, which then promotes contractility and growth cone collapse [70]. Simultaneously, ephexin1 triggers actin depolymerization and growth cone collapse by inhibiting RAC1 and CDC42, which normally function to promote extension of lamellipodia and filapodia [69-72].

EPH forward signaling can also regulate growth cone dynamics through localized inhibition of the mTOR pathway, resulting in decreased protein synthesis in the growth cone [73-75]. Activation by ephrinA1 promotes rapid EPHA phosphorylation and decreases ERK1/2 phosphorylation, resulting in derepression of Tuberous sclerosis (TSC) complexes and inhibition of the mTOR pathway. In mice, RGCs axotomy results in downregulation of mTOR [76], consistent with their limited ability to regenerate. However, constitutive activation of mTOR by knocking out *Tsc1*, *Tsc2* or the mTOR inhibitor *Pten* (phosphatase and tensin homolog) promotes RGC axon outgrowth and regeneration [76]. Likewise, growth cone collapse in rat hippocampal neurons is triggered by EPHA/ephrinA1 activation or by rapamycin, an mTOR inhibitor, and is associated with decreased protein synthesis in growth cones [74, 77]. However, in motor neurons derived from embryonic stem cells, growth cone collapse resulting from ephrinA5 simulation is independent of protein synthesis [78]. Thus, mechanisms regulating growth cone dynamics downstream of EPH/ephrin signaling vary between different neuronal types and likely reflect the integration of a variety of attractive and/or inhibitory cues present in a cell's environment.

4.3. Ephrin Reverse Signaling

Following receptor/ligand binding, both ephrinA and ephrinB are capable of reverse signaling in the ligand bearing cell [19, 79]. Because of their lack of intracellular domains, ephrinAs were not expected to mediate reverse signaling. However, knocking out *EphA7*, which is expressed in the superior colliculus but not in RGCs, results in inappropriate collicular terminations of retinal ganglion cell located in both the ventral and nasal retina, a finding consistent with a loss of ephrinA reverse signaling in the RGCs [80]. In stripe assays using retinal explants from mouse (E15.5-16.5) or chick (E7), nasal RGCs, which express higher levels of ephrinAs and lower levels of EPHAs, do not extend neurites on substrates composed of EPHA7-Fc [80]. This effect was mediated via the ephrinA's present on the RGCs, as blocking ephrinAs on the RGCs by pre-incubation of the explants with soluble EPHA7-Fc abolished the ability of nasal RGC processes to avoid EPHA7-containing substrates [80]. Effects of ephrinA reverse signaling on RGC growth cone dynamics are mediated, in part, through interaction with co-receptors, including the neurotrophin receptors $p75^{NTR}$ and TrkB [81, 82]. Loss of $p75^{NTR}$ in knockout mice results in a loss of sensitivity of nasal RGC axons to EPHA7 *in vitro* and $p75^{NTR}$ knockout mice have defects in the retino-tectal mapping of nasal RGCs *in vivo* [83]. The expression domains of $p75^{NTR}$, ephrinA5 and ephrinA2 overlap on RGCs and EPHA7-Fc simulation increases $p75^{NTR}$/ephrinA2 co-localization [83]. EphrinA5 also associates with TrkB on RGC axons and ephrinA5 overexpression increases BNDF-induced axon branching in the absence of EPHA [82].

EphrinB reverse signaling was first evidenced by the differences in the phenotypes of *EphB2* null mice and mice in which only the *EphB2* extracellular domain was deleted [84]. EphrinB2 reverse signaling was subsequently implicated in formation of topographic maps [83, 85], axon guidance [86], cell migration [87], cell adhesion [88] and retinal vascular development [89]. In the optic tectum of *Xenopus*, ephrinB2 is localized to the presynaptic region of RGC axon terminals and infusion of EPHB2-Fc increases ephrinB2 phosphorylation and increases formation and maturation of RGC synapses [90].

Following receptor binding, ephrinA and ephrinB reverse signaling both activate SRC-family tyrosine kinases in the ligand bearing cells [91-93]. In ephrinA reverse signaling, receptor binding and clustering stimulates signal transduction and protein phosphorylation through AKT, LCK and FYN [54, 92, 94]. In ephrinB reverse signaling, receptor binding and clustering induces phosphorylation of the ephrinB cytoplasmic domains through rapid recruitment of SRC family kinases, including SRC and FYN [91, 95]. Activated ephrinB can also recruit the SRC homology domain adaptor protein, GRB4 [96] and PDZ-RGS3, a regulator of heterotrimeric G-protein coupled signaling [87]. GRB4 interacts with cytoskeletal regulating proteins, including dynamin, the Abl interacting protein-1 (Abi-1) and the Cbl-associated protein (CAP), resulting in redistribution of these proteins away from focal adhesion complexes and reducing cell adhesion [96]. GBR4 also interacts with axin, a highly conserved protein that is best known as a regulator of β-catenin stability in both WNT signaling and at adherens junctions, but is also involved in axon outgrowth and synaptic plasticity [96-99]. PDZ-RGS3 co-localizes with ephrinB to inhibit G-coupled protein signaling and chemotaxis by cerebellar granule cells [87, 100]. EphrinB reverse signaling can be shut off by subsequent recruitment of protein phosphatase containing PTP-BL proteins [91]. However, a full understanding of how the different downstream signal transduction pathways activated by ephrin reverse signaling are integrated to regulate RGC axon pathfinding and retinotectal mapping remains a work in progress.

4.4. EPH/Ephrin Signaling in *cis*

There are cells in the retina, optic tectum/superior colliculus and elsewhere that express both EPH receptors and ephrin ligands. For example, *ephrinA5* is expressed in a nasal high/temporal low gradient that is reciprocal to nasal low/temporal high gradient of EPHA5/EPHA6 and overlaps the uniform expression of EPHA4 in the mouse retina. This creates the potential for *cis* interactions between both EPHA/ephrinA and EPHB/ephrinB class receptors and ligands that are co-expressed on the same cell. A key consequence of *cis*-binding of EPHs and ephrins is to attenuate the cellular response to ephrins that are presented in *trans* by neighboring cells [50, 52, 101]. Thus, EPHs that are expressed uniformly across the retina can be differentially silenced by the gradient of co-expressed ephrins [102]. However, there are questions as to whether this applies across all cell types or for all receptor/ligand pairs, as several studies have found that EPH receptors and EFN ligands are segregated in discrete membrane domains within an individual cell that would preclude *cis*-interactions [50, 51].

4.5. EPH/Ephrin Cleavage and Internalization

Given the relatively high affinities of EPH receptor/EFN ligand binding and the subsequent multimerization of the complexes, EPH/ephrin binding might be predicted to mediate cell-cell adhesion. However, both adhesion and repulsion have been observed following receptor/ligand binding. The differential responses and the termination of EPH/ephrin forward and reverse signaling is modulated, in part, by regulated cleavage and/or internalization of receptors and ligands [53, 103-107]. Receptor phosphorylation, downstream of ligand binding and receptor clustering, is also associated with internalization of the receptor/ligand complex [108]. In primary neuronal cultures from mouse embryonic brain, activation by ephrinB2-FC stimulates cleavage of the extracellular domain of EPHB2 by gamma secretase, which appears to limit EPHB forward signaling and enhance ephrinB reverse signaling. Moreover, both the receptor and the ligand can be internalized by the EPH expressing cells and, in some instances, can involve transcytosis of the entire ligand, including the intracellular domain, along with the EPH receptor. When Swiss T3T fibroblasts overexpressing FLAG-tagged ephrinB2, labeled at the C-terminus of the cytoplasmic domain, contacted cells overexpressing EPHB4, both the EPHB4 and ephrinB2 were detected in vesicles within the EPHB4 expressing cells [109]. However receptor internalization by EPHB4 expressing cells depends on the kinase activity of the EPHB4 receptor, as deletion of the intracellular domain or mutation to generate kinase-dead receptors decreased internalization by the EPHB4 expressing cells and increased internalization by the ephrinB2 expressing cells [109].

Endocytosis of receptor/ligand complexes, either with cleavage (endocytosis) or without cleavage (transcytosis) of the ligand contributes to repulsion and/or growth cone collapse via EHP/ephrin interactions. [110]. However, in neuroblastoma cells, mutations that prevent cleavage of ephrinA3 can block neurite withdrawal, but not growth cone collapse, showing that these are regulated independently [107]. Retinotopic mapping in mice is dependent on endocytosis and overexpression of a modified EPHA8 that is resistant to endocytosis leads to an anterior shift in the termination zones of nasal RGCs, that is the opposite of what is observed following overexpression of an intact EPHA8 [105]. In primary cultures of mouse forebrain neurons, contact between cells that overexpress either EPHB2 or ephrinB1 results in transcytosis and internalization of the entire receptor/ligand complex, including the intracellular domains [104]. The timing of transcytosis by the ephrinB1 expressing cell (reverse signaling) was rapid, whereas the transcytosis by the EPHB2 expressing cell (forward signaling) was slow, suggesting a potential mechanism for the varied cellular responses to ligand/receptor binding. The mechanism for internalization of EPH/ephrin complexes functions via two main pathways: caveoli endocytosis [111], and clathrin mediated endocytosis [112]. Interestingly, endocytosis can either target EPH/ephrin complexes for degradation [103, 109] or can result in recycling the receptors back to the cell surface [113], offering another mechanism to modulate cellular responses to EPH/ephrin signaling.

Caveoli (Latin for little caves) are small (<100 nm) indentations in the plasma membrane that are a specialized type of lipid raft [114]. Caveoli are associated with endocytosis, particularly in the context of signal transduction and over-expression of caveolin, a key structural protein, is sufficient to induce caveoli formation [115]. EPHB1 and EPHA2 receptor are localized in caveoli, and after ligand binding EPHA2 receptors interact with caveolin-1 [111]. Signal transduction downstream of EPHB1 can be blocked by overexpression of mutated caveolin-1 that cannot form polymers or induce caveoli formation [111]. Interestingly, multiple signaling molecules that interact with EPH receptors have also been shown to be localized in caveoli, including other receptor tyrosine kinases (e.g., TRKB, $P75^{NTR}$, EGFR) and components of downstream intracellular signal transduction pathways (e.g., RAS, ERK2, FYN and SRC) [116, 117, 118]. Variability in the types of molecules that are internalized in concert with EPH/ephrin complexes is likely to contribute to the variation in cellular responses to EPH/ephrin signaling.

There is also evidence for EPH/ephrin stimulation of clathrin mediated endocytosis in retinotectal mapping [105]. In HEK293 cells, activation of EPHA8 forward signaling by ephrinA5-Fc results in rapid receptor/ligand internalization in clathrin containing vesicles [106]. Rat B35 neuroblastoma cell that over-express EPHB2 show increased formation of clathrin-coated pits following activation with soluble ephrinB2-Fc [119]. Clathrin-mediated endocytosis is dependent on EPHB2-mediated phosphorylation of synaptojanin, a phosphatidylinositol 5′-phosphatase required for clathrin-mediated endocytosis [119]. Similarly, stimulation of ephrinB1 expressing cells with soluble EPHB1-Fc results in clathrin-mediated endocytosis by the ephrinB1 expressing cell [112]. Interestingly, other tryrosine kinase receptors (e.g., EGF receptors and $P75^{NTR}$) can be internalized by clathrin-mediated instead of caveoli-mediated endocytosis, depending on the ligand [120, 121].

5. EPH/EPHRIN EXPRESSION IN RETINA AND RETINO-RECIPIENT AREAS

In amphibians, teleost fish and birds (e.g., chick) and rodents (e.g., mice), the RGCs primarily project to the optic tectum/superior colliculus where visual input is integrated with other sensory modalities, including auditory and tactile input. In humans, non-human primates and other species with a high degree of visual acuity, the majority of RGCs project to the lateral geniculate nucleus (LGN), with a smaller component terminating in the superior colliculus. To date, the majority of research on Eph/ephrin signaling in the visual system has focused on the retino-tectal/retino-collicular mapping.

Fitting with Sperry's original chemoaffinity model, the generally accepted dogma of Eph/ephrin expression in the retina is that specific *Eph* receptors are expressed in gradients across the nasal/temporal (*EphA*) and dorsal/ventral (*EphB*) axes of the retina during visual system development and their cognate *ephrinA* and *ephrinB* ligands are expressed in reciprocal gradients across the anterior-posterior and medial-lateral axes of optic tectum/superior colliculus respectively (Figure 2) [1, 49, 79]. In fish, chick and mouse, the retinotopic organization of RGC projections to the optic tectum are similar: RGCs located in the nasal retina (low EPHA) terminate in the caudal optic tectum (high EFNA), those in the temporal retina (high EPHA) terminate in the rostral tectum (low EFNA); RGCs located in the dorsal retina (low EPHB) terminate in the lateral optic tectum (low EFNB) and those in the ventral retina (high EPHB) terminate in the medial tectum (high EFNB) [122]. Although the role of *Eph/ephrin* signaling in specification of the retinotopic map is well accepted, the specific EPH and ephrins that contribute to retino/tectal patterning vary between species and some have dynamic patterns of expression. Further, both ephrin receptors and ligands are present in the retina and in retinorecipient areas, further complicating our understanding of their roles. This section will focus on the expression patterns in the retina and retinorecipient areas in several of the major experimental animal models. The evidence supporting a role for EPH/ephrin signaling in retinotopic mapping and in specifying the ipsilateral and contralateral projections will discussed be in Section 6. As noted in the introduction, the gene names of many ephrins and ephrin receptors have changed since their initial identification [123, 124] (Table 1). In this section, many of the original names are included parenthetically at the first usage for a particular species, but the current nomenclature will be used in the text thereafter.

Table 1. Eph receptors and ephrin ligands; nomenclature and retinal expression

Protein	Alternate names	Unigene (retina)	Protein	Alternate names	Unigene (retina)
EPHA1	Eph, Esk	---	EFNA1	B61, LERK-1, EFL-1	---
EPHA2	Eck, Myk2, Sek2	+ (m, h)	EFNA2	ELF-1, CEK7-L LERK-6, zf-ephL3	+ (m, h*)
EPHA3	Cek4, Mek4, Hek, Tyro4, Hek4	+ (m, h)	EFNA3	Ehk1-L, EFL-2 LERK-3	+ (m)
EPHA4	Sek, Sek1 Cek8 Hek8, Tyro1	+ (m, h)	EFNA4	LERK-4, EFL-4	+ (m, h*)
EPHA5	Ehk1, Bsk, Cek7, Hek7, Rek7	+ (m, h)	EFNA5	AL-1, RAGS, EFL-5 LERK-7, ephL4	+ (m, h)
EPHA6	Ehk2, Hek12	---			
EPHA7	Mdk1, Hek11, Ehk3, Ebk, Cek11, zdk1	+ (m, h*)			
EPHA8	Eek, Hek3	+ (m, h)			
EPHA10		+ (m, h)			
EPHB1	Elk, Cek6, Net, Hek6	+ (m, h)	EFNB1	LERK-2, elk-L EFL-3. Cek5-L, STRA-1	+(m, h*)
EPHB2	Cek5, Sek3, Nuk, Erk Tyro5, Hek5, Drt, Qek5	+ (m, h)	EFNB2	Htk-L, ELF-2, LERK-5 NLERK-1	+(m, h)
EPHB3	Cek10, Hek2, Mdk5 Tyro6, Sek4	+ (m, h*)	EFNB3	NLERK-2, Elk-L3 EFL-6 ELF-3, LERK-8	+(m, h*)
EPHB4	Htk, Myk1, Tyro11 Mdk2	+ (h*)			
EPHB5	(removed from Unigene/NCBI database; identical to EPHB6)				
EPHB6	Mep, Cek9, Hek9	+ (m, h)			

+, Unigene database contains clones from retina or eye cDNA libraries from human (h) or mouse (m).

---, no clones reported from retina/eye in Unigene database; *, library source-whole eye.

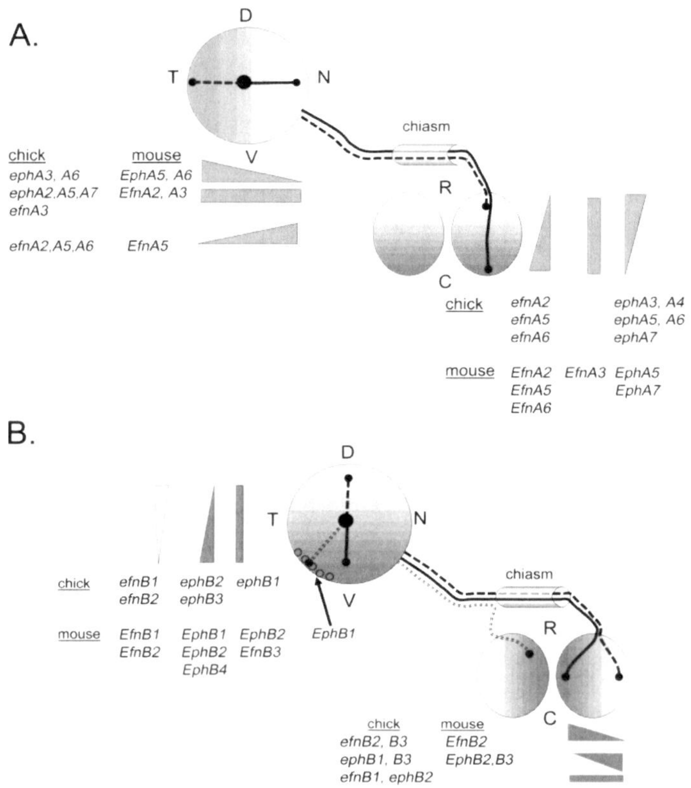

Figure 2. EPH/ephrins in retinotectal mapping.
Diagrams showing orientation of expression gradients of ephrin ligands (*Efn*) and receptors (*Eph*) expression in the retina and optic tectum/superior colliculus in chick and mouse retinas and the spatial mapping of RGC axon terminals. Triangles show orientation of gradients of mRNA expression, with rectangles for uniform expression. Gene names for relevant receptors and ligands from chick and mouse are matched with their expression patterns. (A) RGC axons from nasal retina (low *EphA*; solid line) connect to the contralateral optic tectum/superior colliculus (ovals) and synapse on postsynaptic cells expressing low high levels of *EfnA* ligands. RGCs from temporal retina (high *EphA*; dashed line) also project contralaterally and synapse in the anterior superior colliculus (low *EfnA*). (B) Along the dorsal/ventral retinal axis, axons from RGCs in dorsal retina (low *EphB*, dashed line) synapse in the lateral regions of the contralateral superior colliculus (low *EfnB*); Axons on RGCs in ventral retina (high *EphB*, solid line) synapse in medial regions of the contralateral superior colliculus (high *EfnB*). In mice, axons from RGCs located in the ventrotemporal crescent (small circles; double dashed line) express *EphB1* and are repelled by *EfnB* in the optic chiasm, causing them to project ipsilaterally to the superior colliculus, where they synapse in the anterior lateral superior colliculus. R, rostral; C, caudal; N, nasal; T, temporal; D, dorsal; V, ventral.

5.1. Fish

Sperry's chemoaffinity model was based on the findings from experiments on optic nerve regeneration in goldfish (*Carrasius auretus)*, and subsequently, expression of both *Ephs* and ephrins was detected in the retina and optic tectum in both goldfish and zebrafish (*Danio rerio*). Although the goldfish has long provided an important model for studying retinal and optic nerve regeneration, zebrafish are now the mainstay in studying visual system development in fish. The time-course of embryonic development in zebrafish is rapid and the time from fertilization to hatching is approximately 3 days, depending on temperature [125]. Eye development follows a similar, rapid progression, with the optic primoridum detectable at ~12 hours post fertilization (hpf) (6 somite stage). The optic primoridum subsequently extends laterally from the diencephalon and cavitates to form the optic vesicle [126]. The bilayered optic cup is present by ~19 hpf (14-21 somite stage) and the first postmitotic retinal ganglion cells are observed in a patch in the ventro/nasal retina at 28 hpf [127]. The visual system in zebrafish is functional at hatching (~72 hpf), as evidenced by visually stimulated behaviors such as prey capture [128], visual startle response and optokinetic eye movements [129, 130].

5.1.1. EPH/Ephrin Expression in Zebrafish Retina

zf-ephA7 (*zdk1*) mRNA is first detected in the optic primordium, in the region destined to form the temporal retina. In the early optic cup, *ephA5* (*rtk7*) is expressed in the retina in a dorsotemporal low/ventronasal high distribution [131]. A robust nasal low/temporal high gradient of *ephA7* mRNA is present in the optic cup at 48 hpf [132-134], a timepoint when RGC axons are innervating the optic tectum [125, 126, 135]. Although *ephA4c* (*rtk4*) mRNA is detected at low levels across the retina, it lacks detectible spatial differences in expression [131]. The expression of EPHA receptors in the mature zebrafish retina has not been reported. However, in the mature retinas of goldfish (6-9 cm in length), both EPHA3 and EPHA5 are detected uniformly, albeit weakly, across the retinal ganglion layer by immunofluorescence labeling [136].

B type ephrin receptors are also expressed in the developing retina in zebrafish and *ephB3a* (*zek3*) is expressed in a ventral high/dorsal low pattern beginning in the optic primordium and continuing throughout larval development [133, 137]. At 28 hpf, *ephB2* mRNA is also expressed in a ventral high/dosal low pattern across the optic cup [138, 139]. In contrast, *ephB4a* (*rtk5*) is detected in the optic stalk, but not in the retina, beginning at the 10 somite stage and continuing until at least the 18 somite stage [131].

Several ephrin ligands are expressed in the zebrafish retina in gradients that are reciprocal to their cognate receptors. In the early optic cup (20 somite stage), binding assays using chick EPHA3 receptor probes show a nasal high/temporal low pattern of EFNA ligands, although retinal expression of *efnA2 (ephL3), and efnA5b (ephL4)* mRNA were reported to be undetectable at this stage [140]. By 24 hpf, there is a distinct nasal high/temporal low gradient of *efnA5b* that is primarily in the ganglion cell layer [140, 141]. Both *efnA2* and *efnA5b* are detected in nasal high/temporal low gradients by 72 hpf, a time when the RGC axons have innervated the optic tectum and visual reflexes are functioning [140]. Although *efnA3* is also expressed in the retina, it is uniformly distributed along the nasal temporal axis in retinal ganglion cells and the innermost portion of the nascent inner nuclear layer [140]. *efnB2a* is present in a dorsal high/ventral low gradient across the optic cup at 28 hpf [138, 139].

5.1.2. EPH/Ephrin Expression in Zebrafish Optic Tectum

The expression patterns of ephrin ligands in the optic tectum are consistent with their role in patterning the connectivity of the RGC axons. Between 24-48 hpf, when RGC axons are extending and have begun to innervate the optic tectum, *efnA2*, *efnA3b*, *efnA5a* and *efnA5b* (*zf-EphL2*) are all expressed in rostral low/caudal high gradients that extend to the midbrain/hindbrain boundary [138, 142]. At 72 hours, *efnA3* shows a distinct rostral low/caudal high gradient of mRNA, whereas *efnA5 is* expressed at low levels across the optic tectum with no obvious gradient [140]. Expression at later stages has not been reported for zebrafish, although juvenile goldfish express ephrinA2 in a subset of cells in the optic tectum, but lack a detectable gradient along the rostral and caudal axis [143].

There are fewer studies of ephrinB ligand expression patterns in the developing optic tectum in zebrafish, but all reported a generally rostral low/caudal high pattern. At 19 hpf (early optic cup), *efnB1a* expression is highest just anterior to the midbrain/hindbrain boundary [139]. At this stage, *ephB4a* is present in a rostral low/caudal high gradient across the optic tectum with a distinct stripe of high expression at the diencephalon/midbrain boundary. *efnB3b* is also present detected in the optic tectum at 32 hpf, although no gradient is apparent [138]. At 72 hpf, when tectal cells have already been contacted by RGC axon terminals, *efnB2a* mRNA expression persists in a subset of RGC target cells across the optic tectum, with a greater number of *efnB2a* expressing cells located in the caudal tectum compared to rostral tectum [144]. In juvenile goldfish, *efnB2* mRNA (*in situ* hybridization) and protein (immunoreactivity) continues to be detected a rostral low/caudal high gradient across the optic tectum [145].

5.2. Chick

As in fish, differences in the timing of developmental stages in chick (*Gallus gallus*) can result from variations in temperature. Therefore, embryonic development in the chick is described both in terms of the Hamburger and Hamilton (HH) stages and hours or days post-fertilization (hpf; dpf) [146]. Optic vesicle formation begins at HH 9 (29-33 hpf) and the optic stalk is visible as a constriction between the optic vesicle and brain by HH 11 (40-45 hpf). Lens placode induction and invagination of the optic vesicle to form the optic cup begins during HH 14 (50-53 hpf). The first postmitotic RGCs are located in the central retina, immediately dorsal to the nascent optic disc and differentiation proceeds from central to peripheral [147]. RGCs begin to extend projections following withdrawal from the cell cycle and axons are found in the optic stalk by HH 19 (68-72 hpf) and at the site of the prospective optic chiasm by HH 22-24 (E3.5-4) [148]. Axons begin to decussate at the optic chiasm around E4 [149], with a very small number of ipsilateral projections detected in the optic tract at HH 25 [150]. The initial retinotectal organization of RGC terminals is detectible by E11 and connections are subsequently refined to generate an accurate map by E15 [151].

5.2.1. EPH/Ephrin Expression in Chick Retina

In chick, *ephA3 (Cek4)* mRNA is first detected in the anterior neural plate and by HH 11, *ephA3* is expressed uniformly across the optic vesicle [152, 153]. Following optic cup formation, both *ephA3* and *ephA5 (Cek8)* are present in RGCs in the retina, but only *ephA3* expression shows a nasal low/temporal high gradient [153-156]. Both *ephA1* (*Cek9*) and *ephA4* (*Cek8*) mRNAs are detected in all retinal layers early in retinal development, but do not show graded expression across the nasal/temporal axis [154, 156-158]. As RGCs mature, expression of both *ephA1* and *ephA4* becomes concentrated within the ganglion cell layer [158-160]. Although not expressed in a gradient, EPHA4 is more highly phosphorylated in the nasal retina at E8 [156], suggesting differential signaling in nasal vs. temporal retina. Low levels of *ephA5* (*Cek7*), *ephA6* (*Ehk2*), and *ephA7* (*Cek11*; *Ehk3)*, but not *ephA2*, are also detected in the retina by *in situ* hybridization [152, 156, 161]. Unexpectedly, *ephA7* (*Cek11*) mRNA lacks nasal/temporal differences in expression, but is reported to be differentially expressed along the dorsal ventral axis at E5, with highest levels in the dorsal two thirds of the retina [161].

By *in situ* hybridization, *ephB1* (*Cek6*), *ephB2* (*Cek5*) and *ephB3* (*Cek10*) are also expressed in the retina, with *ephB2* most prominent [156]. In the retina at E7 (~HH stage 30-31), both *ephB2* and *ephB3* are highest in ventral retina, with little mRNA detected in the dorsal retina [156, 157, 162, 163]. EPHB2 protein expression corresponds to reported mRNA patterns and is present in the axons of RGCs that originate from the ventral retina [157, 164]. In contrast, *ephB1* is expressed at low levels, primarily in the ganglion cell layer, but no gradient is reported [163].

EphrinA ligands are also expressed in the chick retina and generally show gradients that are complementary to the patterns of *ephA* receptor expression. EphrinA2 (*Cek7-L*) and ephrinA5 (*RAGS*) mRNA are detected in the anterior neural tube of chick early in development and are detected in the optic vesicles as early as HH stage 10 Baker [152]. At E6 (~HH stage 29), both ephrinA2 and ephrinA5 proteins are detected immunostaining in the nerve fiber layer and GCL, with the nasal low/temporal high pattern of ephrinA2 extending across the retina and ephrinA5 predominantly restricted to the temporal retina [102, 165]. By E8 (~HH stage 34), ephrinA6 protein is robustly detected in all retinal layers in a nasal high/temporal low gradient, whereas weak ephrin5 immunoreactivity is restricted to the ganglion cell and nerve fiber layer in the temporal retina [38].

EphrinB1(*Cek5-L*) mRNA expression is robust in the dorsal retina and shows a dorsal high/ventral low gradient of expression in both RGCs and the inner nuclear layer from E3 (~HH stage 24) to at least E14 [163]. The retinal cells expressing *efnB2* (*elf-2*) are limited to the central-most portion of dorsal retina and are entirely contained within the larger expression domain of *efnB1* [161-163, 166]. By both immunostaining and affinity probes, EFNB1 and EFNB2 proteins are primarily localized to the inner and outer plexiform layers, and are not detected in the optic nerve or in RGC axons [163], suggesting that they may contribute to dendritic connectivity rather than retino-tectal mapping. A different pattern of expression is reported for e*phB5*, which is present in a central low/peripheral high gradient across the retina at E4.5, with lowest levels in the areas where β-tubulin-labeled RGC axons are already projecting to the optic disc [161]. As the central to peripheral wave of

RGC differentiation proceeds, *ephB5* expression recedes, leaving only low levels of *ephB5* mRNA in the most peripheral retinal zones [161]. The timing of the spatial changes in *ephB5* expression suggests a potential contribution in preventing axon outgrowth away from the optic disc, rather than in patterning retinotectal connections.

5.2.2. EPH/Ephrin Expression in Chick Optic Tectum

Expression of *efnA2* (elf-1/ephrin-ligand family 1) in the optic tectum begins around E2 (~HH stage 13) and is robust by E3 (~HH stage 19), prior to innervation by RGC axons [154]. Both ephrinA2 and ephrinA5 (*elf-5*) are detected in rostral low/caudal high gradients by E8 [38, 154, 167-169]. In contrast, ephrinA6 expression is low in the optic tectum at E8 without an obvious gradient of expression along the anterior/posterior axis [38]. By *in situ* hybridization, *efnB1* and *efnB2* are also detected in the optic tectum in chicks, with *efnB1* expressed in gradient that is highest in the medial and lowest in the lateral optic tectum as early as E3 (HH stage ~19) [163, 170]. At E8, the *efnB1* gradient is still detected, with mRNA primarily in the superficial retinorecipient layers, although tectal expression is gone by E14 when retino-tectal mapping is complete. By immunostaining, EFNB1 protein is detected in the radial glia [163] and EPHB2-Fc binding confirms the medial/lateral low distribution of EFNB ligands in the optic tectum. EphrinB2 is also expressed in a gradient, with highest levels in the posterior optic tectum and, at E6-E8, *efnB2* mRNA is primarily located in cells located in the deeper layers that contain output neurons of the tectum, rather than in the retinorecipient layer [156].

In chick, *ephA3* is expressed in multiple brain areas, including the optic tectum, where *ephA3* mRNA is detected a rostral-medial high/caudal-lateral low gradient [153]. Based on intensity of *in situ* staining, the overall levels of *ephA3* mRNA expression appears to be higher in the optic tectum than in the retina [156]. Transcripts for *ephA4* (*Cek8*), *ephA5* (*Cek7*) and *ephA7* (*Cek11*) are detected within a rostral high/caudal low gradient in the *stratum griseum* central, the primary retinorecipient area of the optic tectum, although expression levels are low at E8 [156]. Both *ephA4* and *epha7* are also expressed in gradients in other retinorecipient areas in the chick brain, but the orientation of the gradient varies: in the lateral anterior nucleus, the gradient shows the same rostral high/caudal low orientation as in the optic tectum, whereas in other retinorecipient nuclei in the diencephalon and mesencephalon, the orientation of the *ephA* gradient is rotated, consistent with the retinotopic organization of projections to these nuclei [169].

The B-class ephrin receptors, *ephB1*, *ephB2* and *ephB3,* are also expressed in the optic tectum, with *ephB2* and *ephB3* expressed in a medial high/lateral low gradient [170, 171]. There is uniform expression of *ephB1* mRNA across the developing optic tectum, with highest in layer II, which will give rise to the retinal recipient layer (*stratum griseum central*) and in presumed postmitotic cells near the subventricular zone [156]. Similar to ephrinB2, *ephB2* and *ephB3* mRNAs are more highly expressed in the deeper layers of the optic tectum [157].

5.3. Rodent (Mice/Rats)

The overall pattern of eye development in rodents is similar to that in chick [172]. In mice, strain differences, rather than temperature differences, can subtly affect the timecourse of development. For rats, with their slightly longer gestation time, developmental milestones typically lag by a day or two, although the sequence of events remains consistent. In mice, the optic pits are first seen prior to neural tube closure and definitive optic vesicles extend laterally from the diencephalon by E9. By E11.5, the bilayered optic cup is present and the first retinal ganglion cells are beginning to withdraw from the cell cycle [173, 174]. Based on anterograde labeling, RGC axons enter the optic stalk on E12 and reach the optic chiasm by E13 [175]. Here, they pause prior to decussating to enter the contralateral optic tract at E14. However, projections from the ventrotemporal retina are not detected in the ipsilateral optic tract until E16.5 [176].

5.3.1. EPH/Ephrin Expression in Mouse Retina

At the optic cup stage, both *EphA5* and *EphA6* are expressed in RGCs in a nasal-low/temporal-high gradient, with *EphA5* also expressed in the cells of the inner nuclear layer [177, 178]. Based on reporter expression in mice with targeted replacement of the intracellular domain of *EphA5* (exons 8-13) with β-galactosidase (β-gal), *EphA5* is expressed as early as E9.5 and is higher in the temporal retina compared to the nasal retina, although a distinct gradient across the retina is not initially apparent [179]. As the first retinal ganglion cells begin to withdraw from the cell cycle, *EphA5* driven β-gal is detected in a distinct temporal (high) to nasal (low) pattern in the nascent ganglion cell layer and inner neuroblastic layer that persists throughout embryonic and fetal development [179]. At E13, *EphA6* also is expressed in a distinct nasal low/temporal high gradient, but expression is restricted to the ganglion cell layer [180, 181]. By E17, when RGCs have projected through the optic tract and have begun to arborize in the ventral lateral geniculate nucleus and superior colliculus, the gradient of *EphA5* remains robust in the RGC layer [179, 182, 183]. At P0 and later, there is a period of connection refinement during which the gradients of *EphA5* and *EphA6* expression persists in the ganglion cell layer [177, 184, 185]. In the mouse retina, *EphA3* is also expressed in a nasal low/temporal high gradient. However, it is not expressed in RGCs, but is limited to cells in the neuroblastic layer and, later, to the inner nuclear layer [177, 184]. *EphA7* has not been detected in the mouse retina at any stage of development [132, 186, 187]. In adult rats, there is a gradual decline in overall *EphA* expression and a flattening of the gradient with age [188, 189].

Several studies reported a largely uniform expression of *EphA4* across the ganglion cell layer [177, 190]. However, analysis of heterozygous β-gal-*EphA4* knock-in transgenic mouse showed transient and diffuse expression in the retinal neuroepithelium only at E11.5 and 12.5, with no expression in RGCs [191]. Based on *in situ* hybridization and β-gal expression, there is robust *EphA4* expression in the optic stalk [191]. *EphA4* expression is progressively restricted to the astrocyte precursors, which surround the optic disc, such that by E14.5, *EphA4* is no longer detected in the retina [191, 192]. Although *EphA4* expression is not detected in migrating astrocyte precursors, it is expressed by mature astrocytes along the vitreal surface of the mature retina and in astrocytes that form the boundary between the retina and optic nerve head [191].

In the mouse, *EphB1*, *EphB2*, *EphB4* and *EphB6* are detected in the retina during the period of RGC axon outgrowth. *EphB2* is the first *EphB* receptor to be expressed and is uniformly expressed in both the ganglion cell layer and the neuroblastic layer at E13.5 [193]. By E15.5, a time when RGC axons are crossing at the optic chiasm, but prior to their innervation of the superior colliculus or dLGN, *EphB2* is expressed in the retina in a dorsal low/ventral high gradient [192-194]. *EphB3* and *EphB6* mRNA is also detected in the ganglion cell layer but shows no apparent gradient of expression [192] [195]. *EphB4* is weakly expressed in all retinal layers at E14.5, but with no apparent gradient [170].

Of the *EphB* receptors, *EphB1* has a unique role and is involved more in specification of the ipsilateral pathway than in overall patterning of the retino/tectal maps. Although initial studies reported no gradient of *EphB1* expression in the ganglion cell layer at E14.5 or E16.5 [193], another study revealed a nasal high/temporal low distribution of *EphB1* mRNA at E14.5

[195]. In transgenics heterozygous for a β-gal knock-in to the *EphB1* locus, β-gal expression marks the *EphB1* expressing cells and revealed a complex and changing pattern of expression [192]. *EphB1* driven β-gal expression in the ganglion cell layer begins around E13 in a patch within the dorso/central retina that is gone by E15.5. Interestingly, this is the area where RGCs first begin to differentiate and pioneer axons from this retinal region are the first to reach and decussate at the optic chiasm [175, 196]. A second domain of *EphB1*- β-gal expression is detected at E14 in the ventro/temporal crescent of the retina, in those RGCs that will give rise to the ipsilateral projections [192]. The initial restricted expression of *EphB1* to the ventro/temporal retina progressively expands and by E17, *EphB1* is now expressed across the entire retina. Intriguingly, expression of *EphB1* outside of the ventro/temporal crescent is present in other retinal cells, but not in ganglion cells [192].

There are fewer reports of ephrin ligand expression in the mouse retina, but *EfnA5* (*AL-1/RAGS*) mRNA is detected in both the ganglion cell and the neuroblastic layers of the mouse retina at E17, in a nasal high/temporal low gradient that is reciprocal to *EphA5*/*EphA6* [180]. Two ephrin ligands, ephrinA2 (*ELF-1*) and ephrinA3 (Ehk1-L/Efl-2/Lerk3), are also detected in the retina following birth and are expressed in the ganglion cell layer at P1 by *in situ* hybridization but show a relatively uniform distribution along the nasal/temoral axis [197]. At P0, ephrinB2 is expressed in a shallow gradient (dorsal high/ventral low) and is relatively evenly detected in all retinal layers [170].

5.3.1. EPH/Ephrin Expression in Rodent (Mice/Rats) Superior Colliculus/LGN

Consistent with the chemoaffinity mapping theory, ephrin ligands are also expressed in gradient patterns across the superior colliculus and LGN of rodents, such as mice and rat. In the midbrain of mice, ephrinA2 (ELF-1), ephrinA3 (Ehk1-L/Efl-2/Lerk3) and ephrinA5 (AL-1/RAGS) are expressed. The earliest expression of ephrinA ligands has been detected at E8.5, when, by *in situ* hybridization, *EfnA2* shows high expression along the rostral/caudal axis of the midbrain, with expression extending into the hindbrain [154, 198]. EphrinA5 is detected in a distinctly rostral low/caudal high gradient across the midbrain, with higher expression in the inferior colliculus and rostral cerebellum [167, 199]. EphrinA3 and ephrinA5 are also expressed in the dorsal lateral geniculate nucleus at P0 [197]. By *in situ* hybridization, ephrinA3 is expressed relatively uniformly across the dLGN, but is present at very low levels in the ventral LGN. EphrinA5 is expressed in a dorsal low/ventral high gradient across the dLGN with a similar oriented but less intensely stained gradient in in the vLGN, based on EPHA3-AP binding.

EphrinB expression begins around E15.5 and ephrinB1 mRNA is distributed in a lateral low/medial high gradient primarily at the ventricular zone and the superior colliculus. At E15.5, ephrinB2 expression is strongest in cells at the midline just dorsal to the path taken by RGC axons and in the region where ventrotemporal (*EphB1*-expressing) RGC axons pause and turn to project along the ipsilateral optic tract [192]. EphrinB3 is also reported to be expressed in the optic chiasm at E15.5 in cells located dorsal and posterior to the projecting RGC axons; however, ephrinB1 is not detected in the optic chiasm in mice [192]. At P0, ephrinB1 and ephrinB3 are detected in the midbrain [170]. EphrinB2 is robustly detected at the ventricular zone of the superior colliculus, with expression restricted to cells at the dorsal and ventral midline [170]. In adult mice, there is minimal binding of EPHB3-AP probes in the superior colliculus, although robust binding is detected elsewhere, leading to the conclusion that minimal ephrinB expression persists in the superior colliculus in the adult [200].

At P0/P1, affinity mapping using ephrinA5-AP ligands shows that EPHA receptors are present in the superior colliculus in a rostral high/caudal low gradient [200]. By *in situ* hybridization, *EphA7* shows a graded rostral high/caudal low expression in the SC, with labeled cells located in both superficial and deep lamina [80]. *EphA4* is uniformly expressed along the rostral/caudal axis and is primarily in the superficial laminae [201]. Ligand binding using ephrinB2-AP detects EPHB in the superior colliculus in adult mice, with binding distributed in a rostral high/caudal low gradient that is most prominent in the superficial and intermediate lamina [200]. There was no obvious medial lateral distribution of ephrinB2 binding.

5.4. Ferret

Although the data on EPH/ephrin expression in the ferret *(Mustela putorius furo*) is limited, there is a considerable body of literature on the development of the visual system in the ferret. It is included here because of its potential utility for studying EPH/ephrin signaling during the more complex mapping of RGCs in the lateral geniculate nucleus. In the ferret, the sequence of developmental milestones is the same as in other vertebrates [202] although the timeline is more protracted. The time from fertilization to birth in ferrets is 42 days, with eye opening delayed until 72 days. By E21, the bilayered optic cup is formed and the retina has thickened into a typical pseudostratified neuroepithelium [203]. RGCs are generated beginning at E22 and continuing thru E29 [204]. Axon outgrowth from RGCs is first detected using lipophilic dyes at E24 when some axons have crossed at the optic chiasm [205]. The inner and outer nuclear layers are separated by a distinct outer plexiform layer by P12 [203].

5.4.1. EPH/Ephrin Expression in Ferret Retina

There is a single report describing *EphA* expression in the visual system of the ferret that revealed a pattern of *EphA5* expression in the retina that is distinct from that in mouse [206]. Using EFNA affinity probes to detect all EPHAs, the gradient of EPHA receptor expression at P3 is highest in the central retina and decreases towards the periphery. Ligand binding is most robust in the ganglion cell layer, but also was detected in the outer neuroblastic layer. This pattern was confirmed for *EphA5* by *in situ* hybridization, which showed robust expression in the ganglion cell layer, and a generally central high/peripheral low gradient. Of note, the subset of ganglion cells located in the temporal retina that give rise to the ipsilateral projections expressed the lowest overall levels of *EphA5*. This pattern of *EphA5* expression did not appear to reflect an intrinsic change in nasal/temporal patterning of the retina, as ephrinA5 was detected in the ganglion cell layer in a nasal high/temporal low gradient that is similar to that seen in mouse. Expression of other Eph/ephrins in the ferret retina has not been reported.

5.4.2. EPH/Ephrin Expression in Ferret Superior Colliculus/LGN

In the ferret, visual projections to the superior colliculus follow a pattern similar to that in mice, with axons of RGCs in the nasal retina terminating in the caudal superior colliculus, those from temporal retina terminating in the rostral superior colliculus [207]. In the ferret, there are also significant RGC projections to the dLGN. At P0, the LGN is unlaminated and is innervated by projections from both eyes, although the component from the contralateral eye is larger [208, 209]. At this stage, the ipsilateral and contralateral projections are overlapping in the caudal dLGN although the contralateral projections extend more medially than the ipsilateral projections [208]. However, all projections are still organized according to retinal position with a typical spatial mapping: RGC axons from the nasal retina projecting to the rostral LGN and those from the temporal retina projecting to the caudal LGN [207]. Subsequently, the ipsilateral and contralateral projections segregate to achieve the mature pattern with ipsilateral projections terminating in the superficial (outermost) layer, and contralateral projections terminating in the deeper layer of the dLGN [207, 210]. By postnatal week 4, the dLGN has developed the characteristic laminar cytoarchitecture present in the adult [208].

EphrinA5 is expressed in the dLGN at P3 in a high rostral/low caudal gradient that is superimposed on a second gradient that is higher near the surface and decreases in the deeper layer of the dLGN [206]. During the lamination of the LGN, the matching of EPHA expressing RGC axon terminals to ephrinA expressing postsynaptic targets follows the typical pattern: RGCs expressing the lowest levels of *EphA5* (ipsilateral nasal retina) retain connections in the superficial layer of the dLGN where ephrinA5 is highest; the axons of RGCs with have highest levels of *EphA5* (contralateral temporal retina), segregate to the deeper layer where ephrinA5 expression is lower. Expression of ephrinA5 expression declines and is undetectable by P5, when the lamination of the dLGN is complete. The expression of the B-type ephrins and their receptors in the ferret has not been described.

5.6. Human/Primate

The development of the eye in humans (*Homo sapiens*) and primates follows a similar developmental pattern and morphogenesis of the eye is completed in the first trimester [211, 212]. In humans, by 28 days post fertilization (dpf) (Carnegie Stage 13), the bilateral optic vesicles are detectable and by 32 dpf (Stage 14), the optic vesicle invaginates to form the optic cup. By week 7 (Stage 19), the ventral optic fissure has closed and the eyes begin to rotate from their initial lateral position towards their final frontal orientation. Histogenesis of the retina is prolonged in primates and shows a central to peripheral developmental gradient with central region differentiating earliest. Proliferation in the human retina ceases around 30 weeks of gestation. Ganglion cells differentiate early and in human embryos, the ganglion cell layer is clearly visible at the posterior pole by 35 days gestation. The fovea is detectible in the developing human retina by 10 weeks as an area of thinner retina with a single layer of cone photoreceptors [213]. In macaque, cellular differentiation begins around 27 dpf and continues to around 120 dpf [214]. The specific EPHs and ephrins detected in the human/macaque retinas to date are consistent with those in mouse, although the patterns of expression are different. The different expression patterns in the human and primate retina appear to reflect the frontal orientation and the larger ipsilateral component of the visual pathways.

5.6.1. EPH/Ephrin Expression in Primate Retina

In the human retina, both *EPHA5 and EPHA6* are detected by *in situ* hybridization as early as gestational weeks 9/10 during retinal histogenesis. *EPHA5* is barely detectable in the nasal-peripheral retina, but expression progressively increases across the retina, reaching the highest expression in central retina and then decreasing towards the temporal retinal margin [215]. There is a slight enrichment in the ganglion cell layer at this stage, although mRNA is detected across the entire thickness of the retina. By 19 weeks, *EPHA5* expression is distinctly enriched in the ganglion cell layer in the central retina. *EPHA6* is expressed in a similar high central/low peripheral gradient, but is present exclusively in the ganglion cell layer. Using microarray and quantitative RT-PCR, spatial differences in *EPHA6* mRNA expression evaluated to compare the macula (5 mm diameter centered on fovea) vs. surrounding tissue from human retina at week 19 [216]. Consistent with the gradients detected by *in situ* hybridization, both EPHA5 and EPHA6 expression is highest in macula [217]. The patterns of EPHA5 and EPHA6 protein expression in the macaque retina are similar to reported mRNA expression in human, with EPHA6 expression primarily in the ganglion cell layer and highest expression at the fovea and lowest expression in the nasal retina. The central high/peripheral low gradients EPHA5 and EPHA6 and the counter gradients of ephrinA in the developing human and macaque retinas are consistent with a role in patterning retinocollicular maps.

Unlike in mice, *EPHB1* in human fetal retinas is present in a gradient across the ganglion cell layer [215]. There is, however, only minimal *EPHB1* expression in nasal retina with the staining intensity essentially flat until the midline of central retina. Here, there is a steep increase in *EPHB1* mRNA expression towards the temporal margin creating a distinct gradient. *EPHB1* mRNA expression is higher in the macula than surrounding retina by 50-70% [216-218]. Although by RT-PCR there is a 30-50% decrease in *EPHB2* mRNA at the macula, the overall expression and distribution of *EPHB2* along the dorsal/ventral axis has not been reported.

By RT-PCR, ephrinA1, A3 and A4, but not ephrinA2, are detected in the human fetal retina at 20 weeks gestation [217, 218]. *EFNA5* was detected by *in situ* hybridization at 9, 10 and 18 weeks gestation in a central low/peripheral high gradient that is complementary to *EPHA6* [215]. Both in terms of intensity and the area stained, *EFNA5* mRNA was increased in the nasal retina at earlier ages, but by 19 weeks, staining in the GCL is of similar intensity in both nasal and temporal retina [215]. Expression of ephrinA5, ephrinA1, ephrinA2 and ephrinA3 are all lowest in the macula compared to surrounding retina [218]. By *in situ* hybridization and immunostaining, ephrinA1 and ephrinA4 co-localize with PAX2 in astrocytes in the optic nerve head at 13 weeks gestation (human) and 55 dpf (macaque) [217, 218]. EphrinA1, but not ephrinA4, is also present in the PAX2 expressing cells that encircle the optic nerve head at the retinal margin at these same developmental stages. Expression of ephrinBs in human retina has not been reported.

5.6.2. EPH/Ephrin Expression in Primate Superior Colliculus/LGN

In humans and primates, the major RGC projections are in the retinogeniculate pathway. In addition, because of the frontal orientation of the eye and the large binocular fields, the meridian that divides the nasal and temporal retina also specifies the contralateral and ipsilateral components of the optic nerve. Axons are present in the optic nerve as early as 7 weeks gestation and reach the optic chiasm and brain nuceli during the 8th week and beyond. RGC axons are detected in the dLGN at 20 weeks gestation (human) and although there is not yet any visible cellular lamination of the LGN, RGC axon terminals already segregated into eye-specific layers [219]. Both *EPHA7* and *EFNA5* are expressed in the dLGN in humans as early as 14 weeks gestation [217, 218]. *EPHA7* shows high dorsomedial to low ventrolateral distribution at weeks 14, 17 and 19. At the same stages, *EFNA5* is in a complementary gradient that is lower dorsomedial and higher ventrolateral. The patterns of *EFNA5* and *EPHA7* expression in the dLGN suggests a role in overall topographic mapping, but are not consistent with a major role in patterning the laminar segregation of the ipsilateral and contralateral pathways.

6. EPH/Ephrin in RGC Axon Pathfinding and Retinotectal Mapping

The development of the retinal projections can be broken into several distinct stages. First, RGC axons must project to the optic disc and away from the peripheral retina to exit into the optic stalk/optic nerve through the nascent optic disc. Second, they must know whether to decussate at the optic chiasm or remain ipsilateral before entering the optic tract. Finally, upon reaching retinorecipient regions, they must synapse with the appropriate target cells and establish the initial retinotopic maps. EPH/ephrin signaling has been implicated in each of these steps.

6.1. Intraretinal Pathfinding

Intraretinal pathfinding is mediated by inhibitory signals in the peripheral retina and permissive signals at the optic disc [220-222]. Although Eph/ephrin signaling is most typically associated with retinotectal mapping, EPHB/ephrinB signaling has been implicated in intraretinal axon pathfinding. In chick, *EphB5* is expressed in a peripheral high, central low pattern and expression recedes towards the periphery as RGC differentiation proceeds [161]. Interestingly, mice lacking *EphB2* and/or *EphB3* have intraretinal pathfinding defects in a subset of RGCs whose axons separate from the main bundles and fail to enter the optic nerve head [193]. This appears to function, in part, through reverse signaling via ephrinB ligands, as mutations that only removed the *EphB2* kinase domain, but retained the extracellular ligand binding domain showed fewer intraretinal pathfinding errors [193].

6.2. Optic Chiasm

Within the central nervous system (CNS), neural pathways to and from the brain typically decussate at the midline, such that information for the left side of the body is processed in the right half of the brain and *vice versa*. In animals with laterally placed eyes that have no overlap of visual fields between the two eyes, ganglion cell axons all cross at the optic chiasm to terminate in the contralateral superior colliculus and LGN [223, 224]. Increased visual overlap between the two eyes is associated with increasing amounts of binocular vision and manifests in an increasing proportion of projections that remain ipsilateral. Mice have only a small region of visual overlap and only a subset of RGCs, located in the ventro-temporal crescent of the retina, contribute to their small ipsilateral pathway [196]. Species with frontally placed eyes, such as humans and most predatory species, have a high degree of overlap between the visual fields of the two eyes, which provides the basis for binocular vision and depth perception. In these species, visual information from each retina is transmitted to both sides of the brain such that visual input from the left half of the visual field is processed on the right side of the brain and that from the right half of the visual field is processed in the left side of the brain. This pattern is established by divergence of retinal axons at the chiasm, such that the axons originating from RGCs in the nasal hemi-retinas project contralaterally and axons originating from RGCs in the temporal hemi-retinas project ipsilaterally. In humans, approximately 40% of axons project ipsilaterally [215, 225].

There is strong evidence that EPHB/ephrinB signaling functions in the decision of RGC axons to cross or remain ipsilateral at the optic chiasm. In the mouse retina, *EphB1* mRNA expression is restricted to RGCs within the ventro-temporal retina at the time when RGC axons are reaching the optic chiasm (E13.5-17.5) and ephrinB2 is expressed on cells within the nascent optic chiasm where they provide a repulsive signal to EPHB1 expressing RGC axons [192]. In mice, formation of ipsilateral projections depends on EPHB1 signaling as genetic ablation of *EphB1* reduces the ipsilateral projections by ~43% [192]. *EphB2* appears to make only minor contributions as *EphB1, EphB2* double knockouts have only a slightly greater reduction (~56%) in the number of ipsilaterally projecting axons. In co-cultures, cells from the optic chiasm inhibit neurite outgrowth by RGCs from the ventrotemporal retina, but have less effect on RGCs from dorsal/temporal retina [226]. This is attributable in large part to EPHB/ephrinB signaling, since blocking ephrinB2 ligands on optic chiasm cells using EPHB4-Fc eliminates their inhibitory effect on ventro/temporal RGC axons and decreases the number of ipsilaterally projecting axons [192, 227, 228].

In contrast, zebrafish do not express ephrinB at the optic chiasm at the time when the RGC axons decussate and have no ipsilateral component to the optic tract [229, 230]. Likewise *Xenopus* tadpoles prior to metamorphosis have no ipsilateral projections and ephrinBs are not present in the optic chiasm [230]. However, during metamorphosis, ephrinB2 is up-regulated at the optic chiasm and signals for RGCs to project into either the contralateral or ipsilateral optic tract. Consistent with this, EPHB2 receptors are expressed on in the ventrotemporal retinas of metamorphosing tadpoles by those RGCs that will project ipsilaterally [230, 231]. Overexpression of zebrafish ephrinB2 in the optic chiasm during embryonic development in *Xenopus* causes inappropriate ipsilateral projections, showing that zebrafish ephrinB expression is able to specify ipsilateral projections, although this is not their role *in vivo* [230].

Although the overall pattern of EPHB1 in human differs from mouse, it is consistent with the larger ipsilateral component of the optic projections, rather than a difference in function. In human retina, EPHB1 is most highly expressed on the RGCs in the temporal hemiretina that will form the ipsilateral pathway and is lowest in the nasal retina on the RGCs that form the contralateral pathway [215]. The gradient of *EPHB1* expression that is present across the temporal retina in human retinal development may contribute additional positional information needed for the appropriate spatial orientation of axon terminals from this large ipsilateral component.

6.3. EPHA/Ephrina Regulation of Retinotopic Mapping

EPHA/ephrinA signaling regulates the topographic mapping of RGCs relative to their position along the nasal/temporal axis of the retina in lower vertebrates (e.g., fish, birds) [1, 49, 79]. The overall repellant activity of ephrinA/EPHA signaling on RGC axon outgrowth has been repeatedly demonstrated in stripe assays, wherein RGCs from the temporal retina preferentially extend axons on membranes from the anterior tectum/superior colliculus and avoid membranes from posterior tectum/superior colliculus. These behaviors can be replicated using substrates of purified ephrinA ligands or membranes from cells that overexpress specific ephrinAs [102, 165, 198, 232-235]. The inhibitory effects of posterior tectal membranes on RGCs in the temporal retina appears to result from ephrinA activation of EPHA forward signaling on the RGCs. Overexpression of a dominant negative *EphA3* that blocks forward, but not reverse, EPHA signaling in chick RGCs abolishes their avoidance of posterior tectal membranes [178]. Consistent with a requirement for EPHA forward signaling in temporal RGCs, in transgenic mouse lacking the *EphA5* intracellular domain, RGCs in temporal retina lose their preference for anterior membranes and extend equally well on membranes from anterior or posterior superior colliculus from wild-type mice [178]. This effect was specific effect to the loss of EPHA5 forward signaling in RGCs, as temporal RGC axons from wild-type mice still avoided membranes isolated from the posterior superior colliculus of homozygous *EphA5-β-gal* mice [178].

There is compelling evidence that it is the relative differences in EPHA expression between RGCs that regulates the position of their termination zones in the superior colliculus. In an elegant study, the *Isl2* promoter was used to overexpress *EphA3*, which is not normally expressed in mouse RGCs, in a subset of RGCs scattered across the retina. This increased the level of total EPHA receptors in the Isl2 expressing subset of RGCs relative to adjacent Isl2-negative RGCs [177]. Focal DiI application in the retina of *Isl2-EphA3* transgenics labeled two termination zones: one in the expected location and the other terminating more rostrally, reflecting the increased EPHA levels in the *Isl2-EphA3* expressing cells. This is consistent with an additive mechanism whereby the total number of EPHA receptors present on a growth cone can determine its response to an ephrinA repulsive signal.

There are reciprocal gradients of EPHAs and EFNAs in both the retina and superior colliculus. As some of the EPHA receptors and EFNA ligands are expressed uniformly across the retina or the colliculus, there are cells that express both receptors and ligands. There is evidence that ephrinA in the nasal retina directly contributes to nasal RGCs' insensitivity to the repellant activities of caudal tectal membranes. Removing all GPI linked ephrinAs from chick RGC axons using phospholipase-C makes nasal axons behave more like temporal axons and avoid substrates of caudal tectal membranes in stripe assays [102]. Conversely, when *EfnA5* is overexpressed on temporal RGCs, they are no longer repelled by membranes from caudal tectum in stripe assays, but instead behave more like nasal axons with no preference for rostral vs. caudal tectal stripes [102]. Consistent with this, retroviral over-expression of ephrinA2 or ephrinA5 in developing chick retinas results in errors in the topographic position of axon terminals from both nasal and temporal RGCs *in vivo* [102, 165]. These findings show that ephrinAs on RGCs actively participate in patterning the retino-tectal mapping of RGCs. The ability of ephrinAs expressed in RGCs to block growth cone collapse that typically results from activation of EPHA forward signaling is likely to be attributable, at least in part, to inhibition of EPHA forward signaling by *cis*-interactions between EPHA and EFNAs co-expressed on RGCs. In HEK293 cells that constitutively overexpress *EphA3*, treatment with ephrinA5-Fc induces receptor phosphorylation, but this effect is blocked by prior transfection of the receptor expressing cells with ephrinA5 expression vectors [101]. When overexpressed in retinal ganglion cells, both EPHA3 and ephrinA3 colocalize to RGC growth cones, supporting the potential for *cis*-interactions [101]. However, on the axons of spinal cord neurons *in vivo*, EPH receptors and their ligands are segregated in discrete membrane domains that would preclude *cis*-interactions [50, 51]. Whether EPHA receptors and ephrin ligands are co-localized or segregated on RGC axons and growth cones when they are present at physiological concentrations *in vivo* remains an open question.

In addition to inhibition of EPHA forward signaling via *cis* interactions between EPHAs/EFNAs on RGCs, reverse signaling through ephrinA ligands plays a role in retinotectal mapping. In mouse, reverse signaling stimulated by the rostral high/caudal low gradient of *EphA7* in the optic tectum is required for correct retinotopic mapping of retinal ganglion cells from the nasal retina [80]. *EphA7* is not expressed in RGCs, but is present in the superior colliculus in a rostral high/caudal low gradient. In *EphA7* knockout mice, axons of RGC in the nasal retina form ectopic arborizations in the superior colliculus [80]. However, nasal axons from both wild-type and *EphA7* knockout mice avoid stripes of EPHA7-Fc *in vitro,* showing that it is the lack of EphA7 in the superior colliculus that alters the patterns of RGC connectivity as a result of the reduction/loss of ephrinA reverse signaling in nasal RGCs.

Reverse signaling through ephrinAs is also associated with brain derived neurotophic factor (BDNF) signaling in RGCs. BDNF is a well-known neurotrophin that promotes neurite outgrowth, branching and arborization of RGC terminals, as well as RGC survival [236]. BDNF signals through high affinity TRK receptors and through the low affinity p75 neurotrophin receptor ($p75^{NTR}$). RGCs express $p75^{NTR}$ and pharmacological inhibition of $p75^{NTR}$ or absence of $p75^{NTR}$ in knockout mice promotes survival of axotomized RGCs [237-239]. In addition to its role in RGC survival, $p75^{NTR}$ is implicated in regulation of axonal branching [81]. The $p75^{NTR}$ is closely associated with ephrinA5 on RGC axons and physically interacts with the ephrinA5 cysteine rich domain [82]. Expression of both ephrinA and $p75^{NTR}$ is required for EPHA repulsion of ephrinA expressing axons [81, 83]. BDNF enhances the ability of ephrinA5 promote axonal branching of chick RGCs *in vitro* and this effect is lost by EPHA7-Fc treatment [82]. The link between ephrinAs and $p75^{NTR}$ provides an intriguing mechanism for integrating different signal transduction cascades that affect RGCs during formation of the retinotectal maps. BDNF is also under investigation as a potential therapeutic agent for treatment of RGC degenerative disease [240, 241]. Therefore it will be important to understand how these two pathways interact in models of RGC injury.

Clearly EPH/ephrin signaling does not function in isolation and other cellular mechanisms contribute to axon pathfinding and the generation of the mature retinotopic maps *in vivo.* The matching of RGC numbers to post-synaptic targets through RGC programmed cell death is part of normal development [242]. Likewise, spontaneous waves of retinal activity function to refine the initial retinotopic maps through the strengthening of synapses of RGCs that fire together and elimination of inappropriate connections [243]. The relative simplicity of the retinotopic maps in lower vertebrates and rodents make them particularly attractive for modeling. Multiple computational approaches have been generated to model the how EPH/ephrin signaling regulates retinotopic map formation [244, 245] and how this fits with the contributions of competition and spontaneous retinal activity in generating the final organization of retinotopic maps [246-248]. The most recent models have begun to integrate contributions of forward and reverse signaling, as well as *cis*-inhibition, on the initial mapping and subsequent stabilization of the retinotectal maps [249, 250]. As we increase our understanding of how eph/ephrin signaling integrates forward and reverse signaling with *cis*-mediated inhibition and other signals, such BDNF/p75^{NTR} signaling, in the relatively simpler models of retinocollicular mapping such as mouse and chick, it will be interesting to apply these models to understand the patterns of connectivity in more complex visual systems in humans at the levels of the lateral geniculate nucleus and beyond.

7. EPH/Ephrin Signaling in RGC Injury and Disease

Understanding the mechanisms that guide the extension and connectivity of RGCs is a key question of developmental biology that is made more urgent by recent advances in stem cell biology and spinal cord regeneration. Currently there are no cures for neurodegenerative diseases that affect the optic nerve including glaucoma, optic neuritis and optic atrophy. For patients with these diseases, pharmacological interventions that can stop progression are unable to restore vision lost as a result of RGC death. Thus, the development of regenerative therapies offers the prospect of restoring lost vision. Although there has been progress in regeneration of other types of retinal neurons from stem cells [251-254], the challenges developing cell-replacement strategies to treat optic neuropathies are daunting. These include not only identifying strategies to regenerate all classes of RGCs from stem cells and to promote axon outgrowth, but it will be critical to understand how to pattern the connectivity following regeneration. For functional vision, the retinotopic maps of RGC connections must be re-established. Thus continued efforts to understand the functions of EPH/ephrin signaling in normal development and disease and the regulatory mechanisms that pattern their expression will be critical for the eventual success of regenerative medicine.

7.1. EPHs/Ephrins in Optic Nerve Regeneration in Fish

In fish, the retina grows continuously, with the new RGCs generated at the retinal margin connecting in the optic tectum [255, 256]. Fish are also capable of regenerating the retina and optic nerve following injury [255-259]. Indeed, this regenerative capacity was the basis of Sperry's experiments leading to the chemoaffinity theory. The ability of regenerating RGC axons to re-connect to the correct topographic location within the optic tectum in fish demonstrates that they possess the positional information necessary for retinotopic mapping. Thus, it was rather unexpected that the gradients of *ephA* expression in the mature retinas of goldfish are less steep than those in the embryonic retina [136]. Similarly, in rats, expression of *EphA5* persists in RGCs, but is reduced compared to the embryonic retina [260]. However, Eph/ephrin receptor expression in the retina changes following optic nerve crush in fish [136, 145, 261] and rat [188, 260]. During optic nerve regeneration in fish, retinal expression of both *ephA3* and *ephA5* is up-regulated and a robust nasal low/temporal high gradient is reestablished

Topographic mapping of RGCs also relies on appropriate expression of ephrin ligands in the brain. Following optic nerve crush and the subsequent deafferentation of the optic tectum in goldfish, the number of ephrinA2 expressing neurons in the caudal optic tectum increases compared to the rostral tectum, [136]. This pattern is maintained during optic nerve regeneration, but by 3 months post-injury after the connections have been re-established, ephrinA expression in the tectum declines [136, 143, 145]. EPHA/ephrinA signaling is required to reestablish the retinotectal mapping of RGCs and blocking EPHA forward signaling by intracranial infusion of soluble EPHA3 decreases the number of ephrinA2 expressing neurons leading to a loss of the gradient of ephrinA2 expression in the optic tectum [145]. Importantly, EPHA/ephrinA signaling is critical for patterning the connectivity of regenerated RGCs and blocking EPHA forward signaling in RGCs results in increased RGC projections to the posterior tectum [145].

7.2. EPHs/Ephrins in Retinal and Optic Nerve Injury in Mammals

In mammals, the optic nerve does not spontaneous regenerate following retinal or optic nerve injury. There are many factors contributing to the lack of regenerative ability, including inhibitory myelin and chondroitin sulfate proteoglycans in the optic nerve and an intrinsic decline in the ability of RGCs to extend axons [220]. However, even after these obstacles are overcome, changes in *Eph/Efn* expression following injury may interfere with successful re-establishment of retinotopic mapping. In the adult rat, optic nerve transaction down-regulates *EphA5* expression in surviving RGCs, particularly those in temporal retina, resulting in a loss of the nasal low/temporal high gradient [188]. Localized laser injuries, which ablate ipsilaterally projecting neurons in the ventro/temporal retina, result in up-regulation of *EphA5* in the nasal RGCs, whereas ablation of contralaterally projecting RGCs in dorso/nasal retina does not alter overall retinal *EphA5* expression [260]. Similarly in mice, optic nerve injury, and the resulting deafferentation of the superior colliculus, does not alter the normal rostral low/caudal high gradient ephrinA expression in the retina [200]. Interestingly, when a peripheral nerve graft was used to promote RGC survival and outgrowth, the gradient of *EphA5* in the rat retina was preserved [145]. This suggests that following injury, rescued RGCs in the mammalian retina are capable of responding to external signals and can upregulate appropriate patterns of *EphA5* expression that would enable them to respond appropriately to topographic cues. Of note, although expression of ephrinA2 in the rat superior colliculus declines with age, ephrinA2 is up-regulated in the superior colliculus following deafferentation by optic nerve transection and a rostral-low/caudal-high gradient is again detected. Interestingly, unilateral retinal injuries result in bilateral retinal increases in *EphA5*, pointing to the existence of retrograde or intraocular signals regulating injury-induced gene expression [260]. Together, these data suggest that at least some of the positional information needed for retinotopic mapping persists in retinorecipient areas following optic nerve injury, although RGC axons may need additional signals to upregulate expression of receptors necessary to reconnect appropriately once axonal regeneration can be achieved.

7.3. EPHs/Ephrins in Glaucoma

Glaucoma is a neurodegenerative optic neuropathy characterized by progressive RGC loss that is associated with increased intraocular pressure [262]. Pharmacological treatment to lower pressure can slow progression of the degeneration, but RGC loss prior to diagnosis and treatment results in permanent visual deficits. Recent studies using animal models and human cell culture have suggested a role for EPH/EFN signaling in glaucoma. In a genome wide transcriptome analysis, genes related to *EPH/EFN* signaling were overrepresented as differentally expressed in primary leukocytes from patients with and without definitive primary open angle glaucoma [263].

There are several reports of expressional patterns of EPHA/EFNA in glaucomatous retina and optic nerve. EphrinA5 is down-regulated in the ganglion cell layer in laser induced ocular hypertension in rats [264]. In the *DBA/2J* mouse model of pigment dispersion glaucoma, a 4-fold decrease in ephrinA5 was reported in the ganglion cell layer at 8 months (when there is significant RGC loss) vs. 3 months (prior to RGC loss) [265]. There are also reports of changes in EPHB/ephrinB expression in different models of experimental ocular hypertension/glaucoma. Following laser-induced glaucoma in rhesus monkeys, expression of ephrinB1 increased in the retina in the retinal astrocytes, Müller glia and RGCs and *EphB1* increased in RGCs [266]. In a separate study using a rat model of laser induced ocular hypertension, ephrinB3 expression increased in the retina [267]. Expression of ephrinB2 is also increased in the ganglion cell layer in *DBA/2J* mice at 8 months vs. 2 months [265]. However, other studies have not reported changes in of *Eph* or ephrin mRNA expression in the retinas of DBA/2J mouse [268] or in laser induced ocular hypertension in rat [269] and monkey [270].

In the optic nerve head in rhesus monkeys with laser-induced glaucoma, double immunolabeling showed increased ephrinB1 and ephrinB2 immunoreactivity in astrocytes and perivascular cells at the optic nerve head in glaucomatous eyes [266]. EphrinB1 and ephrinB2 are up-regulated by 12-fold in astroctyes isolated from glaucomatous human donor eyes compared to astrocytes from age matched, non-glaucomatous retinas [271]. Similar increases in *EphB2* mRNA and ephrinB2 mRNA have been reported in DBA/2J mice at 9 months, and double immunolabeling localized the increased EPHB2 expression to macrophages (MOMA2$^+$) and ephrinB2 expression to astrocytes (GFAP$^+$) and microglia (IBA-1$^+$) [272]. In mice with laser-induced hypertension, mRNA expression of *EphB1*, *EphB2* and ephrinB3 is also increased in a subset of astrocytes and microglia in the optic nerve head [273].

There are differences in the reported changes in gene expression between different animal models and some studies have not detected changes in expression of Ephs or ephrins, making it difficult to identify a specific role for EPH/ephrin signaling in glaucoma. However, there is evidence that EPHB signaling contributes to axonal protection. Following laser induced ocular hypertension *EphB2* or *EphB3* knockout mice have respective increases in axonal loss of 21% and 28%, compared to wild type mice [274]. In this study, they also tested the consequences of ocular hypertension on axon loss in *EphB2-β-gal* mice that lack only the cytoplasmic domain of EPHB2, but retain a functional extracellular ligand binding domain. These mice show an intermediate phenotype, with more surviving axons than the *EphB2* null mice but still greater axonal loss than wild-type mice [274]. Since the presence of the extracellular domain in the *EphB2-β-gal* mice is sufficient for activating reverse signaling through the EFNB ligands, these findings show that both forward and reverse EPHB signaling contribute to axonal survival. Consistent with this, when retinas (with optic nerves attached) from wild type mice with laser induced ocular hypertension were cultured in the presence of EPHB2-Fc, there was an 80% increase in β-III tubulin immunoreactivity in the retina, consistent with axon preservation by activation of EPHB/ephrinB reverse signaling [274]. The consistent up-regulation of EPHB and ephrinB expression in retinal and optic nerve astrocytes and in macrophages and microglia within the optic nerve head and suggests a possible role for glia in axonal protection. Since astrocytes are in direct contact with RGC axons in the nerve fiber layer and optic nerve head, they are positioned to initiate signaling via EPH receptors and ligands.

8. Regulation of EPH Receptor Expression in the Retina

Although the role of *Eph/ephrin* signaling in formation of retinotopic maps is well established, the molecular mechanisms that regulate *Eph* expression in the retina are less well understood. A microarray analysis of genes that are differentially expressed in the dorsal, nasal, ventral or temporal mouse retina at E14.5 did not report any transcription factors that were differentially expressed [181]. Using a variety of *in vivo*, *in vitro* and genetic approaches, several transcription factors have been identified as potential regulators of *Eph* receptors in the retina, although evidence supporting direct regulation through binding at the promoters is less robust. There is some evidence for modulation of *Eph* expression by epigenetic mechanisms. In addition, differential phosphorylation or protein trafficking may contribute to post-translational regulation of EPH receptor function. This section focuses on what is known about transcriptional regulation of *Eph* receptor expression in the retina. For a review on regulation outside of the retina, readers are referred to a recent review [275].

8.1. Regulation of EPHAs by Fox and Hmx Transcription Factors

In chick, the winged-helix transcription factors *foxG1*(CBF1) and *foxD1* (CBF2) are respectively expressed in the nasal and temporal halves of the optic vesicle and presumptive optic stalk as early as HH stage 9 [155]. In mice there is a similar distribution, with *FoxG1* in the nasal hemiretina and optic stalk and *FoxD1* in the temporal retina and optic stalk [180, 276]. There is good evidence for mutual repression, as overexpression of *foxG1* in the temporal retina decreases *foxD1* expression [155, 277] and overexpression of *foxD1* in nasal retina represses *foxG1* [278]. In chick, overexpression of *foxD1* up-regulates *ephA3* leading to inappropriate projections of nasal RGCs to the rostral tectum; conversely, overexpression of *foxG1* reduces expression of *ephA4* and results in defects in trajectory of temporal RGCs to the caudal tectum [155, 278, 279]. In *FoxD1* knockout mice, expression of both *EphA5* and *EphA6* is reduced in the temporal retina [180]. Consistent with this, temporal axons lose their topographic specificity and by-pass the rostral tectum to terminate in the caudal portion of the tectum, resulting in a mis-wired pattern of connectivity [180].

Similar to *foxD1*, homeobox containing transcription factors, *hmx1* (*GH6*) and *hmx*-related *SOHo1* are also expressed in nasal high/temporal low patterns in the developing chick optic cup at HH stage 14/15 with the overall expression pattern reciprocal to the gradient of *ephA3* [153]. A similar nasal high/temporal low distribution of *Hmx1* transcripts is in zebrafish and mice in the optic cup [280, 281]. However, no ortholog of chick *SOHo1* has been reported in mammals. Retroviral misexpression studies in chick place *hmx1* and SOHo1 upstream of *ephA3*, as overexpression of either *hmx1* or *SOHo1* blocked *ephA3* expression in RGCs [153]. However, *hmx1* or *SOHo1* overexpression had no effect on the expression patterns of ephrinA5, *ephB2* or *ephA4* in developing retina or on *ephA3*, ephrinA2 or ephrinA5 in the optic tectum. Overexpression of *hmx1* or *SOHo1* resulted in targeting errors of RGCs along the rostral caudal axis of the optic tectum, consistent with the downregulation of *ephA3* [153]. It is interesting to note that in zebrafish, *hmx1* knockdown results in microphthalmia, delayed RGC differentiation and a variety of extraocular defects [281]. Mutations in *Hmx1* cause microphthalmia in mice, although these animals showed few additional phenotypes apart from defects in the formation of the external ear [282]. In humans, mutations in *HMX1* have been identified in patients with Oculo-Auricular syndrome [283]. This genetic disorder affects primarily the eyes and ears and, in the retina, patients typically manifest a variety of defects including microophthalmia, coloboma, cod-cone dystrophy, nystagmus and a sunken, cone-shaped optic disc resembling morning glory syndrome [284]. Although these findings show that HMX1 has functions beyond a role in anterior/posterior patterning in the retina, it would be interesting to determine if the optic disc defect and/or nystagmus in patients with HMX1 mutations are related to defects in the axonal projections of RGCs.

Based on these and other findings, Takahashi and colleagues [278] proposed a model for transcriptional regulation upstream of *ephA3*, *efnA3* and *efnA5* in the chick retina. This model proposes that expression of *foxG1* and *foxD1* is modulated by FGF signaling which specifies an anterior identity and by WNT signaling which promotes a posterior identity within the optic vesicle. These initial signals result in non-uniform expression of *foxG1* and *foxD1* along the anterior/posterior axis, and enables mutual repression to establish restricted domains of expression in the nasal (*foxG1*) and temporal (*foxD1*) optic vesicle/optic cup. *FoxD1* in the temporal retina subsequently represses *hmx1* and *SOHo1*, leading to derepression of *ephA3* expression in temporal retina. Because *foxG1* functions primarily as a repressor, its ability to activate expression of ephrinA2 and ephrinA5 most likely relies on repression of as yet unknown intermediary(s) to relieve inhibition of ephrinA2 and ephrinA5 in the nasal retina.

8.2. Regulation of EPHB1 by Zic2

There is good evidence for regulation of *EphB1* by *Zic2*. The transcription factor *Zic2* is expressed in the ventral/temporal crescent from E13.5-17.5, specifically in the cells that give rise to the small ipsilateral projections in mice [285]. In *Xenopus* tadpoles, both before and after metamorphosis, in albino and pigmented mouse and in the ferret, the extent of *Zic2* expression correlates with the size of the ipsilateral pathways [285]. Since the RGCs that form the ipsilateral component of the optic tract express *EphB1* [192], it is not unexpected that the *Zic2* expressing cells are also *EphB1* positive [228, 285, 286]. Transgenic mice with reduced expression of *Zic2* have fewer axons in their ipsilateral projections [285], a phenotype similar to that of E*phB1* knockout mice [228]. Co-expression reflects a regulatory role for *Zic2* and loss of *Zic2* down-regulates *EphB1* expression [285]. Over-expression of *Zic2* in RGCs that normally decussate results in up-regulation *EphB1* and induces these RGCs to avoid ephrinB2 containing substrate and to project into the ipsilateral optic tract [228, 287]. *Zic2* also regulates an *EphB1* independent pathway in specification of ipsilateral retinal projections, as mis-expression of *Zic2* in *EphB1* knockout mice also increases the number of ipsilateral projections, although not to wild-type levels [228].

8.3. Regulation by WNT Signaling

Regulation of *EphA* receptor expression by WNT signaling has been proposed based in part on the role of WNT signaling in axis formation during embryonic development [288] and on the effects of WNT3a on *FoxD1/FoxG1* expression in chick [277]. Although this would suggest an indirect role for WNT signaling in *Eph* transcriptional regulation, WNT signaling has recently been directly implicated in RGC axon guidance in the midbrain, where WNT3 is expressed by cells in a medial high/lateral low gradient in both chick optic tectum and mouse superior colliculus [289]. Cell membranes from WNT3 overexpressing cells stimulated neurite outgrowth from dorsal but not ventral RGCs and this effect is abolished by blocking antibodies against the WNT receptor, RYK [289]. *Ryk* is expressed in RGCs in a low dorsal/high ventral gradient across the retina in both chick and mice during early development, consistent with a role in regulating retinotectal mapping [289]. Although overexpression of dominant negative RYK in developing chick retina broadened the termination zones towards the midline, the expression patterns of *ephB2* and *efnB2* were not changed. Thus, WNT/RYK signaling may modulate EPHB/ephrinB signaling during topographic mapping of RGC axon terminals in the tectum, but it does not appear to function through direct regulation of *ephB2* or *efnB2* expression.

However, a more direct role for WNT signaling in regulating expression or function of other ephrin receptors and ligands cannot be ruled out. Canonical WNT signaling regulates transcription by activation of TCF/Lef transcription factors [290-292] and multiple *Eph* and *Efn* promoters contain conserved TCF/Lef binding sites [18, 29]. In addition, disheveled (*Dsh*) is a downstream effector of WNT signaling that participates in stabilizing β-catenin in canonical WNT signaling and also contributes to WNT-RYK and WNT-calcium intracellular signaling [293]. In *Xenopus* embryos, DSH is recruited to both EPHBs and ephrinBs following receptor/ligand binding, through interactions with SH adaptor proteins GBR4 and/or NCK [294]. This results in activation of RHOA signaling leading to the repulsive cues necessary for segregation of neural progenitors during embryonic segmentation and is independent of WNT activation of canonical or planar cell polarity pathways. Whether similar signal integration occurs in retinal/tectal mapping in higher vertebrates remains an unanswered question.

8.4. Regulation of by DNA Methylation

Epigenetic modification of genomic DNA through CpG methylation and histone tail modifications represent additional mechanisms of gene regulation that are involved in the dynamic regulation of cell specific genes during neuronal development [295]. Many of the key developmental genes that specify cell fate contain promoters with regions of high CpG density that are regulated by CpG methylation [296]. *Eph* receptor genes all contain phyologenetically conserved CpG islands near their promoters and are candidates for regulation by DNA methylation. Silencing of *EphA* and *EphB* gene expression by DNA hypermethylation has been demonstrated in a variety of cancers [297-305]. In promoter activation/luciferase assays, transcriptional activity of mouse *EphA5* promoter constructs can be blocked by hypermethylation of all CpG dinucleotides [306]. Conversely, in a mouse retinal cell line derived from Müller glia, global DNA demethylation using 5-aza-2-deoxycytidine reverses *EphA5* promoter hypermethylation resulting in re-expression of *EphA5* [306].

More intriguing is the finding that in the mouse retina at P0, there is a subtle increase in CpG methylation near the *EphA5* transcription start site in the nasal retina and activity of promoter constructs can be increased or decreased by different patterns of partial methylation [306]. Similar changes in methylation were not detected for *EphB1* or *EphB2* in any retinal quadrant, suggesting this finding may not be generalizable to all *Eph* receptor genes expressed in the retina. These findings do point to the potential for small variations in promoter methylation to modulate the spatial differences in *EphA5* expression. Sites of increased methylation in the *EphA5* promoter included predicted binding sites for SP/KLF family transcription factors. Combined with the report that overexpression of KLF transcription factors can alter neurite outgrowth by RGCs [307], this large family of transcriptional regulators are potential regulators of *EphA5* in the retina.

Conclusion

The relative simplicity of the retinotopic maps in lower vertebrates and rodents make them particularly attractive for modeling how EPH/ephrin signaling regulates retinotopic map formation [245, 246, 248, 250, 308-310]. Clearly EPH/ephrin signaling does not function in isolation and other mechanisms contribute to axon pathfinding and the generation of the mature retinotopic maps *in vivo*. These include not only other guidance molecules present in the visual pathways, but also the matching of RGC numbers to post-synaptic targets through RGC programmed cell death as part of normal development [242] and the refinement of retinotopic maps through spontaneous waves of retinal activity [243, 311]. Integrating all of these factors into a unified model will continue to challenge researchers in the field. A robust model could prove valuable in understanding the more complex visual system in humans and how EPH/ephrin signaling contributes to the complex patterns of connectivity in the LGN and visual cortex.

Continued research is needed to expand our knowledge of EPH/ephrin signaling in the context of retinal and optic nerve degeneration, to identify strategies to modulate EPH/ephrin expression and to better understand how EPH/ephrin signaling is integrated with other signal transduction cascades. A complete understanding of the contributions and mechanisms of EPH/ephrin signaling in RGC connectivity has potential to contribute to the development novel therapeutic strategies to promote axonal survival, decrease axonal degeneration and/or eliminate inhibitory cues for axon regrowth.

REFERENCES

[1] Cang, J and Feldheim, DA, Developmental mechanisms of topographic map formation and alignment. *Annu Rev Neurosci*, 2013. 36, 51-77.

[2] Wain, HM, Bruford, EA, Lovering, RC, Lush, MJ, Wright, MW, and Povey, S, Guidelines for human gene nomenclature. *Genomics*, 2002. 79, 464-470.

[3] Maltais, LJ, Blake, JA, Chu, T, Lutz, CM, Eppig, JT, and Jackson, I, Rules and guidelines for mouse gene, allele, and mutation nomenclature: A condensed version. *Genomics*, 2002. 79, 471-474.

[4] Sperry, RW, Chemoaffinity in the orderly growth of nerve fiber patterns and connections. *Proc Natl Acad Sci U S A*, 1963. 50, 703-710.

[5] Sharma, SC and Ungar, F, Histogenesis of the goldfish retina. *J Comp Neurol*, 1980. 191, 373-382.

[6] Gaze, RM and Keating, MJ, The visual system and "neuronal specificity". *Nature*, 1972. 237, 375-378.

[7] Barbera, AJ, Marchase, RB and Roth, S, Adhesive recognition and retinotectal specificity. *Proc Natl Acad Sci U S A*, 1973. 70, 2482-2486.

[8] Gottlieb, DI, Rock, K and Glaser, L, A gradient of adhesive specificity in developing avian retina. *Proc Natl Acad Sci U S A*, 1976. 73, 410-414.

[9] Trisler, D and Collins, F, Corresponding spatial gradients of top molecules in the developing retina and optic tectum. *Science*, 1987. 237, 1208-1209.

[10] Constantine-Paton, M, Blum, AS, Mendez-Otero, R and Barnstable, CJ, A cell surface molecule distributed in a dorsoventral gradient in the perinatal rat retina. *Nature*, 1986. 324, 459-462.

[11] McLoon, SC, A monoclonal antibody that distinguishes between temporal and nasal retinal axons. *J Neurosci*, 1991. 11, 1470-1477.

[12] Stahl, B, Muller, B, von Boxberg, Y, Cox, EC and Bonhoeffer, F, Biochemical characterization of a putative axonal guidance molecule of the chick visual system. *Neuron*, 1990. 5, 735-743.

[13] Bonhoeffer, F and Huf, J, In vitro experiments on axon guidance demonstrating an anterior-posterior gradient on the tectum. *EMBO J*, 1982. 1, 427-431.

[14] Walter, J, Kern-Veits, B, Huf, J, Stolze, B and Bonhoeffer, F, Recognition of position-specific properties of tectal cell membranes by retinal axons in vitro. *Development*, 1987. 101, 685-696.

[15] Hirai, H, Maru, Y, Hagiwara, K, Nishida, J and Takaku, F, A novel putative tyrosine kinase receptor encoded by the eph gene. *Science*, 1987. 238, 1717-1720.

[16] Drescher, U, Eph family functions from an evolutionary perspective. *Curr Opin Genet Dev*, 2002. 12, 397-402.

[17] Mellott, DO and Burke, RD, The molecular phylogeny of eph receptors and ephrin ligands. *BMC Cell Biol*, 2008. 9, 27.

[18] Katoh, M and Katoh, M, Comparative integromics on eph family. *Int J Oncol*, 2006. 28, 1243-1247.

[19] Xu, NJ and Henkemeyer, M, Ephrin reverse signaling in axon guidance and synaptogenesis. *Semin Cell Dev Biol*, 2012. 23, 58-64.

[20] Singh, A, Winterbottom, E and Daar, IO, Eph/ephrin signaling in cell-cell and cell-substrate adhesion. *Front Biosci (Landmark Ed)*, 2012. 17, 473-497.

[21] Salvucci, O and Tosato, G, Essential roles of ephb receptors and ephrinb ligands in endothelial cell function and angiogenesis. *Adv Cancer Res*, 2012. 114, 21-57.

[22] Hruska, M and Dalva, MB, Ephrin regulation of synapse formation, function and plasticity. *Mol Cell Neurosci*, 2012. 50, 35-44.

[23] Chen, Y, Fu, AK and Ip, NY, Eph receptors at synapses: Implications in neurodegenerative diseases. *Cell Signal*, 2012. 24, 606-611.

[24] Brantley-Sieders, DM, Clinical relevance of ephs and ephrins in cancer: Lessons from breast, colorectal, and lung cancer profiling. *Semin Cell Dev Biol*, 2012. 23, 102-108.

[25] Himanen, JP, Ectodomain structures of eph receptors. *Semin Cell Dev Biol*, 2012. 23, 35-42.

[26] Hock, B, Bohme, B, Karn, T, Yamamoto, T, Kaibuchi, K, Holtrich, U, ... Strebhardt, K, Pdz-domain-mediated interaction of the eph-related receptor tyrosine kinase ephb3 and the ras-binding protein af6 depends on the kinase activity of the receptor. *Proc Natl Acad Sci U S A*, 1998. 95, 9779-9784.

[27] Smalla, M, Schmieder, P, Kelly, M, Ter Laak, A, Krause, G, Ball, L, ... Oschkinat, H, Solution structure of the receptor tyrosine kinase ephb2 sam domain and identification of two distinct homotypic interaction sites. *Protein Sci*, 1999. 8, 1954-1961.

[28] Stapleton, D, Balan, I, Pawson, T and Sicheri, F, The crystal structure of an eph receptor sam domain reveals a mechanism for modular dimerization. *Nat Struct Biol*, 1999. 6, 44-49.

[29] Katoh, Y and Katoh, M, Comparative integromics on ephrin family. *Oncol Rep*, 2006. 15, 1391-1395.

[30] Nikolov, D, Li, C, Lackmann, M, Jeffrey, P and Himanen, J, Crystal structure of the human ephrin-a5 ectodomain. *Protein Sci*, 2007. 16, 996-1000.

[31] Nikolov, DB, Li, C, Barton, WA and Himanen, JP, Crystal structure of the ephrin-b1 ectodomain: Implications for receptor recognition and signaling. *Biochemistry*, 2005. 44, 10947-10953.

[32] Himanen, JP, Saha, N and Nikolov, DB, Cell-cell signaling via eph receptors and ephrins. *Curr Opin Cell Biol*, 2007. 19, 534-542.

[33] Lackmann, M, Oates, AC, Dottori, M, Smith, FM, Do, C, Power, M, ... Boyd, AW, Distinct subdomains of the epha3 receptor mediate ligand binding and receptor dimerization. *J Biol Chem*, 1998. 273, 20228-20237.

[34] Labrador, JP, Brambilla, R and Klein, R, The n-terminal globular domain of eph receptors is sufficient for ligand binding and receptor signaling. *EMBO J*, 1997. 16, 3889-3897.

[35] Xu, K, Tzvetkova-Robev, D, Xu, Y, Goldgur, Y, Chan, YP, Himanen, JP, and Nikolov, DB, Insights into eph receptor tyrosine kinase activation from crystal structures of the epha4 ectodomain and its complex with ephrin-a5. *Proc Natl Acad Sci U S A*, 2013. 110, 14634-14639.

[36] Blits-Huizinga, CT, Nelersa, CM, Malhotra, A and Liebl, DJ, Ephrins and their receptors: Binding versus biology. *IUBMB Life*, 2004. 56, 257-265.

[37] Pabbisetty, KB, Yue, X, Li, C, Himanen, JP, Zhou, R, Nikolov, DB, and Hu, L, Kinetic analysis of the binding of monomeric and dimeric ephrins to eph receptors: Correlation to function in a growth cone collapse assay. *Protein Sci*, 2007. 16, 355-361.

[38] Menzel, P, Valencia, F, Godement, P, Dodelet, VC and Pasquale, EB, Ephrin-a6, a new ligand for epha receptors in the developing visual system. *Dev Biol*, 2001. 230, 74-88.

[39] Qin, H, Noberini, R, Huan, X, Shi, J, Pasquale, EB, and Song, J, Structural characterization of the epha4-ephrin-b2 complex reveals new features enabling eph-ephrin binding promiscuity. *J Biol Chem*, 2010. 285, 644-654.

[40] Guo, FY and Lesk, AM, Sizes of interface residues account for cross-class binding affinity patterns in eph receptor-ephrin families. *Proteins*, 2013.

[41] Himanen, JP, Chumley, MJ, Lackmann, M, Li, C, Barton, WA, Jeffrey, PD, ... Nikolov, DB, Repelling class discrimination: Ephrin-a5 binds to and activates ephb2 receptor signaling. *Nat Neurosci*, 2004. 7, 501-509.

[42] Brambilla, R, Bruckner, K, Orioli, D, Bergemann, AD, Flanagan, JG, and Klein, R, Similarities and differences in the way transmembrane-type ligands interact with the elk subclass of eph receptors. *Mol Cell Neurosci*, 1996. 8, 199-209.

[43] Gale, NW, Holland, SJ, Valenzuela, DM, Flenniken, A, Pan, L, Ryan, TE, ... Yancopoulos, GD, Eph receptors and ligands comprise two major specificity subclasses and are reciprocally compartmentalized during embryogenesis. *Neuron*, 1996. 17, 9-19.

[44] Sakano, S, Serizawa, R, Inada, T, Iwama, A, Itoh, A, Kato, C, ... Suda, T, Characterization of a ligand for receptor protein-tyrosine kinase htk expressed in immature hematopoietic cells. *Oncogene*, 1996. 13, 813-822.

[45] Bowden, TA, Aricescu, AR, Nettleship, JE, Siebold, C, Rahman-Huq, N, Owens, RJ, ... Jones, EY, Structural plasticity of eph receptor a4 facilitates cross-class ephrin signaling. *Structure*, 2009. 17, 1386-1397.

[46] Egea, J and Klein, R, Bidirectional eph-ephrin signaling during axon guidance. *Trends Cell Biol*, 2007. 17, 230-238.

[47] Pasquale, EB, Eph receptors and ephrins in cancer: Bidirectional signalling and beyond. *Nat Rev Cancer*, 2010. 10, 165-180.

[48] Scicolone, G, Ortalli, AL and Carri, NG, Key roles of ephs and ephrins in retinotectal topographic map formation. *Brain Res Bull*, 2009. 79, 227-247.

[49] Triplett, JW and Feldheim, DA, Eph and ephrin signaling in the formation of topographic maps. *Semin Cell Dev Biol*, 2012. 23, 7-15.

[50] Kao, TJ and Kania, A, Ephrin-mediated *cis*-attenuation of eph receptor signaling is essential for spinal motor axon guidance. *Neuron*, 2011. 71, 76-91.

[51] Marquardt, T, Shirasaki, R, Ghosh, S, Andrews, SE, Carter, N, Hunter, T, and Pfaff, SL, Coexpressed epha receptors and ephrin-a ligands mediate opposing actions on growth cone navigation from distinct membrane domains. *Cell*, 2005. 121, 127-139.

[52] Yin, Y, Yamashita, Y, Noda, H, Okafuji, T, Go, MJ, and Tanaka, H, Epha receptor tyrosine kinases interact with co-expressed ephrin-a ligands in *cis*. *Neurosci Res*, 2004. 48, 285-296.

[53] Janes, PW, Nievergall, E and Lackmann, M, Concepts and consequences of eph receptor clustering. *Semin Cell Dev Biol*, 2012. 23, 43-50.

[54] Davy, A, Gale, NW, Murray, EW, Klinghoffer, RA, Soriano, P, Feuerstein, C, and Robbins, SM, Compartmentalized signaling by gpi-anchored ephrin-a5 requires the fyn tyrosine kinase to regulate cellular adhesion. *Genes Dev*, 1999. 13, 3125-3135.

[55] Bruckner, K, Pablo Labrador, J, Scheiffele, P, Herb, A, Seeburg, PH, and Klein, R, Ephrinb ligands recruit grip family pdz adaptor proteins into raft membrane microdomains. *Neuron*, 1999. 22, 511-524.

[56] Campbell, TN, Davy, A, Liu, Y, Arcellana-Panlilio, M and Robbins, SM, Distinct membrane compartmentalization and signaling of ephrin-a5 and ephrin-b1. *Biochem Biophys Res Commun*, 2008. 375, 362-366.

[57] Shenoy-Scaria, AM, Dietzen, DJ, Kwong, J, Link, DC and Lublin, DM, Cysteine3 of src family protein tyrosine kinase determines palmitoylation and localization in caveolae. *J Cell Biol*, 1994. 126, 353-363.

[58] Robbins, SM, Quintrell, NA and Bishop, JM, Myristoylation and differential palmitoylation of the hck protein-tyrosine kinases govern their attachment to membranes and association with caveolae. *Mol Cell Biol*, 1995. 15, 3507-3515.

[59] Gauthier, LR and Robbins, SM, Ephrin signaling: One raft to rule them all? One raft to sort them? One raft to spread their call and in signaling bind them? *Life Sci*, 2003. 74, 207-216.

[60] Wimmer-Kleikamp, SH, Janes, PW, Squire, A, Bastiaens, PI and Lackmann, M, Recruitment of eph receptors into signaling clusters does not require ephrin contact. *J Cell Biol*, 2004. 164, 661-666.

[61] Mann, F, Miranda, E, Weinl, C, Harmer, E and Holt, CE, B-type eph receptors and ephrins induce growth cone collapse through distinct intracellular pathways. *J Neurobiol*, 2003. 57, 323-336.

[62] Holland, SJ, Gale, NW, Gish, GD, Roth, RA, Songyang, Z, Cantley, LC, ... Pawson, T, Juxtamembrane tyrosine residues couple the eph family receptor ephb2/nuk to specific sh2 domain proteins in neuronal cells. *EMBO J*, 1997. 16, 3877-3888.

[63] Hock, B, Bohme, B, Karn, T, Feller, S, Rubsamen-Waigmann, H, and Strebhardt, K, Tyrosine-614, the major autophosphorylation site of the receptor tyrosine kinase hek2, functions as multi-docking site for sh2-domain mediated interactions. *Oncogene*, 1998. 17, 255-260.

[64] Etienne-Manneville, S and Hall, A, Rho gtpases in cell biology. *Nature*, 2002. 420, 629-635.

[65] Elowe, S, Holland, SJ, Kulkarni, S and Pawson, T, Downregulation of the ras-mitogen-activated protein kinase pathway by the ephb2 receptor tyrosine kinase is required for ephrin-induced neurite retraction. *Mol Cell Biol*, 2001. 21, 7429-7441.

[66] Dail, M, Richter, M, Godement, P and Pasquale, EB, Eph receptors inactivate r-ras through different mechanisms to achieve cell repulsion. *J Cell Sci*, 2006. 119, 1244-1254.

[67] Miao, H, Strebhardt, K, Pasquale, EB, Shen, TL, Guan, JL, and Wang, B, Inhibition of integrin-mediated cell adhesion but not directional cell migration requires catalytic activity of ephb3 receptor tyrosine kinase. Role of rho family small gtpases. *J Biol Chem*, 2005. 280, 923-932.

[68] Murai, KK and Pasquale, EB, New exchanges in eph-dependent growth cone dynamics. *Neuron*, 2005. 46, 161-163.

[69] Shamah, SM, Lin, MZ, Goldberg, JL, Estrach, S, Sahin, M, Hu, L, ... Greenberg, ME, Epha receptors regulate growth cone dynamics through the novel guanine nucleotide exchange factor ephexin. *Cell*, 2001. 105, 233-244.

[70] Sahin, M, Greer, PL, Lin, MZ, Poucher, H, Eberhart, J, Schmidt, S, ... Greenberg, ME, Eph-dependent tyrosine phosphorylation of ephexin1 modulates growth cone collapse. *Neuron*, 2005. 46, 191-204.

[71] Nobes, CD and Hall, A, Rho, rac and cdc42 gtpases: Regulators of actin structures, cell adhesion and motility. *Biochem Soc Trans*, 1995. 23, 456-459.

[72] Gauthier-Rouviere, C, Vignal, E, Meriane, M, Roux, P, Montcourier, P, and Fort, P, Rhog gtpase controls a pathway that independently activates rac1 and cdc42hs. *Mol Biol Cell*, 1998. 9, 1379-1394.

[73] Wang, X and Proud, CG, The mtor pathway in the control of protein synthesis. *Physiology (Bethesda)*, 2006. 21, 362-369.

[74] Nie, D, Di Nardo, A, Han, JM, Baharanyi, H, Kramvis, I, Huynh, T, ... Sahin, M, Tsc2-rheb signaling regulates epha-mediated axon guidance. *Nat Neurosci*, 2010. 13, 163-172.

[75] Sahin, M, Eph receptor and mtor pathway crosstalk: Implications for cancer. *Cell Cycle*, 2010. 9, 2053-2054.

[76] Park, KK, Liu, K, Hu, Y, Smith, PD, Wang, C, Cai, B, ... He, Z, Promoting axon regeneration in the adult cns by modulation of the pten/mtor pathway. *Science*, 2008. 322, 963-966.

[77] Abe, N, Borson, SH, Gambello, MJ, Wang, F and Cavalli, V, Mammalian target of rapamycin (mtor) activation increases axonal growth capacity of injured peripheral nerves. *J Biol Chem*, 2010. 285, 28034-28043.

[78] Nedelec, S, Peljto, M, Shi, P, Amoroso, MW, Kam, LC, and Wichterle, H, Concentration-dependent requirement for local protein synthesis in motor neuron subtype-specific response to axon guidance cues. *J Neurosci*, 2012. 32, 1496-1506.

[79] Feldheim, DA and O'Leary, DD, Visual map development: Bidirectional signaling, bifunctional guidance molecules, and competition. *Cold Spring Harb Perspect Biol*, 2010. 2, a001768.

[80] Rashid, T, Upton, AL, Blentic, A, Ciossek, T, Knoll, B, Thompson, ID, and Drescher, U, Opposing gradients of ephrin-as and epha7 in the superior colliculus are essential for topographic mapping in the mammalian visual system. *Neuron*, 2005. 47, 57-69.

[81] Poopalasundaram, S, Marler, KJ and Drescher, U, Ephrina6 on chick retinal axons is a key component for p75(ntr)-dependent axon repulsion and trkb-dependent axon branching. *Mol Cell Neurosci*, 2011. 47, 131-136.

[82] Marler, KJ, Becker-Barroso, E, Martinez, A, Llovera, M, Wentzel, C, Poopalasundaram, S, ... Drescher, U, A trkb/ephrina interaction controls retinal axon branching and synaptogenesis. *J Neurosci*, 2008. 28, 12700-12712.

[83] Lim, YS, McLaughlin, T, Sung, TC, Santiago, A, Lee, KF, and O'Leary, DD, P75(ntr) mediates ephrin-a reverse signaling required for axon repulsion and mapping. *Neuron*, 2008. 59, 746-758.

[84] Henkemeyer, M, Orioli, D, Henderson, JT, Saxton, TM, Roder, J, Pawson, T, and Klein, R, Nuk controls pathfinding of commissural axons in the mammalian central nervous system. *Cell*, 1996. 86, 35-46.

[85] Wallace, MM, Kavianpour, SM and Gabriele, ML, Ephrin-b2 reverse signaling is required for topography but not pattern formation of lateral superior olivary inputs to the inferior colliculus. *J Comp Neurol*, 2013. 521, 1585-1597.

[86] Bush, JO and Soriano, P, Ephrin-b1 regulates axon guidance by reverse signaling through a pdz-dependent mechanism. *Genes Dev*, 2009. 23, 1586-1599.

[87] Lu, Q, Sun, EE, Klein, RS and Flanagan, JG, Ephrin-b reverse signaling is mediated by a novel pdz-rgs protein and selectively inhibits g protein-coupled chemoattraction. *Cell*, 2001. 105, 69-79.

[88] Arvanitis, DN, Behar, A, Tryoen-Toth, P, Bush, JO, Jungas, T, Vitale, N, and Davy, A, Ephrin b1 maintains apical adhesion of neural progenitors. *Development*, 2013. 140, 2082-2092.

[89] Salvucci, O, Maric, D, Economopoulou, M, Sakakibara, S, Merlin, S, Follenzi, A, and Tosato, G, Ephrinb reverse signaling contributes to endothelial and mural cell assembly into vascular structures. *Blood*, 2009. 114, 1707-1716.

[90] Lim, BK, Matsuda, N and Poo, MM, Ephrin-b reverse signaling promotes structural and functional synaptic maturation in vivo. *Nat Neurosci*, 2008. 11, 160-169.

[91] Palmer, A, Zimmer, M, Erdmann, KS, Eulenburg, V, Porthin, A, Heumann, R, ... Klein, R, Ephrinb phosphorylation and reverse signaling: Regulation by src kinases and ptp-bl phosphatase. *Mol Cell*, 2002. 9, 725-737.

[92] Holen, HL, Shadidi, M, Narvhus, K, Kjosnes, O, Tierens, A, and Aasheim, HC, Signaling through ephrin-a ligand leads to activation of src-family kinases, akt phosphorylation, and inhibition of antigen receptor-induced apoptosis. *J Leukoc Biol*, 2008. 84, 1183-1191.

[93] Coate, TM, Swanson, TL and Copenhaver, PF, Reverse signaling by glycosylphosphatidylinositol-linked manduca ephrin requires a src family kinase to restrict neuronal migration in vivo. *J Neurosci*, 2009. 29, 3404-3418.

[94] Huai, J and Drescher, U, An ephrin-a-dependent signaling pathway controls integrin function and is linked to the tyrosine phosphorylation of a 120-kda protein. *J Biol Chem*, 2001. 276, 6689-6694.

[95] Holland, SJ, Gale, NW, Mbamalu, G, Yancopoulos, GD, Henkemeyer, M, and Pawson, T, Bidirectional signalling through the eph-family receptor nuk and its transmembrane ligands. *Nature*, 1996. 383, 722-725.

[96] Cowan, CA and Henkemeyer, M, The sh2/sh3 adaptor grb4 transduces b-ephrin reverse signals. *Nature*, 2001. 413, 174-179.

[97] Luo, W and Lin, SC, Axin: A master scaffold for multiple signaling pathways. *Neurosignals*, 2004. 13, 99-113.

[98] Chen, Y, Fu, AK and Ip, NY, Axin: An emerging key scaffold at the synapse. *IUBMB Life*, 2013. 65, 685-691.

[99] Stamos, JL and Weis, WI, The beta-catenin destruction complex. *Cold Spring Harb Perspect Biol*, 2013. 5, a007898.

[100] Lu, Q, Sun, EE and Flanagan, JG, Analysis of pdz-rgs3 function in ephrin-b reverse signaling. *Methods Enzymol*, 2004. 390, 120-128.

[101] Carvalho, RF, Beutler, M, Marler, KJ, Knoll, B, Becker-Barroso, E, Heintzmann, R, ... Drescher, U, Silencing of epha3 through a *cis* interaction with ephrina5. *Nat Neurosci*, 2006. 9, 322-330.

[102] Hornberger, MR, Dutting, D, Ciossek, T, Yamada, T, Handwerker, C, Lang, S, ... Drescher, U, Modulation of epha receptor function by coexpressed ephrina ligands on retinal ganglion cell axons. *Neuron*, 1999. 22, 731-742.

[103] Fasen, K, Cerretti, DP and Huynh-Do, U, Ligand binding induces cbl-dependent ephb1 receptor degradation through the lysosomal pathway. *Traffic*, 2008. 9, 251-266.

[104] Zimmer, M, Palmer, A, Kohler, J and Klein, R, Ephb-ephrinb bi-directional endocytosis terminates adhesion allowing contact mediated repulsion. *Nat Cell Biol*, 2003. 5, 869-878.

[105] Yoo, S, Kim, Y, Noh, H, Lee, H, Park, E, and Park, S, Endocytosis of epha receptors is essential for the proper development of the retinocollicular topographic map. *EMBO J*, 2011. 30, 1593-1607.

[106] Yoo, S, Shin, J and Park, S, Epha8-ephrina5 signaling and clathrin-mediated endocytosis is regulated by tiam-1, a rac-specific guanine nucleotide exchange factor. *Mol Cells*, 2010. 29, 603-609.

[107] Hattori, M, Osterfield, M and Flanagan, JG, Regulated cleavage of a contact-mediated axon repellent. *Science*, 2000. 289, 1360-1365.

[108] Pitulescu, ME and Adams, RH, Eph/ephrin molecules--a hub for signaling and endocytosis. *Genes Dev*, 2010. 24, 2480-2492.

[109] Marston, DJ, Dickinson, S and Nobes, CD, Rac-dependent trans-endocytosis of ephrinbs regulates eph-ephrin contact repulsion. *Nat Cell Biol*, 2003. 5, 879-888.

[110] Litterst, C, Georgakopoulos, A, Shioi, J, Ghersi, E, Wisniewski, T, Wang, R, ... Robakis, NK, Ligand binding and calcium influx induce distinct ectodomain/gamma-secretase-processing pathways of ephb2 receptor. *J Biol Chem*, 2007. 282, 16155-16163.

[111] Vihanto, MM, Vindis, C, Djonov, V, Cerretti, DP and Huynh-Do, U, Caveolin-1 is required for signaling and membrane targeting of ephb1 receptor tyrosine kinase. *J Cell Sci*, 2006. 119, 2299-2309.

[112] Parker, M, Roberts, R, Enriquez, M, Zhao, X, Takahashi, T, Pat Cerretti, D, ... Chen, J, Reverse endocytosis of transmembrane ephrin-b ligands via a clathrin-mediated pathway. *Biochem Biophys Res Commun*, 2004. 323, 17-23.

[113] Boissier, P, Chen, J and Huynh-Do, U, Epha2 signaling following endocytosis: Role of tiam1. *Traffic*, 2013. 14, 1255-1271.

[114] Lajoie, P and Nabi, IR, Lipid rafts, caveolae, and their endocytosis. *Int Rev Cell Mol Biol*, 2010. 282, 135-163.

[115] Le, PU, Guay, G, Altschuler, Y and Nabi, IR, Caveolin-1 is a negative regulator of caveolae-mediated endocytosis to the endoplasmic reticulum. *J Biol Chem*, 2002. 277, 3371-3379.

[116] Couet, J, Sargiacomo, M and Lisanti, MP, Interaction of a receptor tyrosine kinase, egf-r, with caveolins. Caveolin binding negatively regulates tyrosine and serine/threonine kinase activities. *J Biol Chem*, 1997. 272, 30429-30438.

[117] Wu, C, Butz, S, Ying, Y and Anderson, RG, Tyrosine kinase receptors concentrated in caveolae-like domains from neuronal plasma membrane. *J Biol Chem*, 1997. 272, 3554-3559.

[118] Gottlieb-Abraham, E, Shvartsman, DE, Donaldson, JC, Ehrlich, M, Gutman, O, Martin, GS, and Henis, YI, Src-mediated caveolin-1 phosphorylation affects the targeting of active src to specific membrane sites. *Mol Biol Cell*, 2013. 24, 3881-3895.

[119] Irie, F, Okuno, M, Pasquale, EB and Yamaguchi, Y, Ephrinb-ephb signalling regulates clathrin-mediated endocytosis through tyrosine phosphorylation of synaptojanin 1. *Nat Cell Biol*, 2005. 7, 501-509.

[120] Henriksen, L, Grandal, MV, Knudsen, SL, van Deurs, B and Grovdal, LM, Internalization mechanisms of the epidermal growth factor receptor after activation with different ligands. *PLoS ONE*, 2013. 8, e58148.

[121] Deinhardt, K, Reversi, A, Berninghausen, O, Hopkins, CR and Schiavo, G, Neurotrophins redirect p75ntr from a clathrin-independent to a clathrin-dependent endocytic pathway coupled to axonal transport. *Traffic*, 2007. 8, 1736-1749.

[122] Lemke, G and Reber, M, Retinotectal mapping: New insights from molecular genetics. *Annu Rev Cell Dev Biol*, 2005. 21, 551-580.

[123] Committee, EN, Unified nomenclature for eph family receptors and their ligands, the ephrins. . *Cell*, 1997. 90, 403-404.

[124] Lemke, G, A coherent nomenclature for eph receptors and their ligands. *Mol Cell Neurosci*, 1997. 9, 331-332.

[125] Kimmel, CB, Ballard, WW, Kimmel, SR, Ullmann, B and Schilling, TF, Stages of embryonic development of the zebrafish. *Dev Dyn*, 1995. 203, 253-310.

[126] Schmitt, EA and Dowling, JE, Early eye morphogenesis in the zebrafish, brachydanio rerio. *J Comp Neurol*, 1994. 344, 532-542.

[127] Hu, M and Easter, SS, Retinal neurogenesis: The formation of the initial central patch of postmitotic cells. *Dev Biol*, 1999. 207, 309-321.

[128] Bianco, IH, Kampff, AR and Engert, F, Prey capture behavior evoked by simple visual stimuli in larval zebrafish. *Front Syst Neurosci*, 2011. 5, 101.

[129] Mueller, KP and Neuhauss, SC, Quantitative measurements of the optokinetic response in adult fish. *J Neurosci Methods*, 2010. 186, 29-34.

[130] Portugues, R and Engert, F, The neural basis of visual behaviors in the larval zebrafish. *Curr Opin Neurobiol*, 2009. 19, 644-647.

[131] Cooke, JE, Kemp, HA and Moens, CB, Epha4 is required for cell adhesion and rhombomere-boundary formation in the zebrafish. *Curr Biol*, 2005. 15, 536-542.

[132] Taneja, R, Thisse, B, Rijli, FM, Thisse, C, Bouillet, P, Dolle, P, and Chambon, P, The expression pattern of the mouse receptor tyrosine kinase gene mdk1 is conserved through evolution and requires hoxa-2 for rhombomere-specific expression in mouse embryos. *Dev Biol*, 1996. 177, 397-412.

[133] Bovenkamp, DE and Greer, PA, Degenerate pcr-based cloning method for eph receptors and analysis of their expression in the developing murine central nervous system and vasculature. *DNA Cell Biol*, 2001. 20, 203-213.

[134] Xu, Q, Alldus, G, Macdonald, R, Wilkinson, DG and Holder, N, Function of the eph-related kinase rtk1 in patterning of the zebrafish forebrain. *Nature*, 1996. 381, 319-322.

[135] Burrill, JD and Easter, SS, Jr., The first retinal axons and their microenvironment in zebrafish: Cryptic pioneers and the pretract. *J Neurosci*, 1995. 15, 2935-2947.

[136] King, CE, Wallace, A, Rodger, J, Bartlett, C, Beazley, LD, and Dunlop, SA, Transient up-regulation of retinal epha3 and epha5, but not ephrin-a2, coincides with re-establishment of a topographic map during optic nerve regeneration in goldfish. *Exp Neurol*, 2003. 183, 593-599.

[137] Thisse, C and Thisse, B, High throughput expression analysis of zf-models consortium clones. *ZFIN Direct Data Submission*, 2005. http://zfin.org.

[138] Erickson, T, French, CR and Waskiewicz, AJ, Meis1 specifies positional information in the retina and tectum to organize the zebrafish visual system. *Neural Dev*, 2010. 5, 22.

[139] Chan, J, Mably, JD, Serluca, FC, Chen, JN, Goldstein, NB, Thomas, MC, ... Roberts, TM, Morphogenesis of prechordal plate and notochord requires intact eph/ephrin b signaling. *Dev Biol*, 2001. 234, 470-482.

[140] Brennan, C, Monschau, B, Lindberg, R, Guthrie, B, Drescher, U, Bonhoeffer, F, and Holder, N, Two eph receptor tyrosine kinase ligands control axon growth and may be involved in the creation of the retinotectal map in the zebrafish. *Development*, 1997. 124, 655-664.

[141] Gosse, NJ, Nevin, LM and Baier, H, Retinotopic order in the absence of axon competition. *Nature*, 2008. 452, 892-895.

[142] Picker, A, Brennan, C, Reifers, F, Clarke, JD, Holder, N, and Brand, M, Requirement for the zebrafish mid-hindbrain boundary in midbrain polarisation, mapping and confinement of the retinotectal projection. *Development*, 1999. 126, 2967-2978.

[143] King, C, Lacey, R, Rodger, J, Bartlett, C, Dunlop, S, and Beazley, L, Characterisation of tectal ephrin-a2 expression during optic nerve regeneration in goldfish: Implications for restoration of topography. *Exp Neurol*, 2004. 187, 380-387.

[144] Wagle, M, Grunewald, B, Subburaju, S, Barzaghi, C, Le Guyader, S, Chan, J, and Jesuthasan, S, Ephrinb2a in the zebrafish retinotectal system. *J Neurobiol*, 2004. 59, 57-65.

[145] Rodger, J, Vitale, PN, Tee, LB, King, CE, Bartlett, CA, Fall, A, ... Beazley, LD, Epha/ephrin-a interactions during optic nerve regeneration:

Restoration of topography and regulation of ephrin-a2 expression. *Mol Cell Neurosci*, 2004. 25, 56-68.

[146] Hamburger, V and Hamilton, HL, A series of normal stages in the development of the chick embryo. *Journal of Morphology*, 1951. 88, 49-92.

[147] McCabe, KL, Gunther, EC and Reh, TA, The development of the pattern of retinal ganglion cells in the chick retina: Mechanisms that control differentiation. *Development*, 1999. 126, 5713-5724.

[148] Navascues, J, Rodriguez-Gallardo, L, Garcia-Martinez, V, Alvarez, IS and Martin-Partido, G, Extra-axonal environment and fibre directionality in the early development of the chick embryo optic chiasm: A light and scanning electron microscopic study. *J Neurocytol*, 1987. 16, 299-310.

[149] Drenhaus, U and Rager, G, Formation of alternating tiers in the optic chiasm of the chick embryo. *Anat Rec*, 1994. 240, 555-571.

[150] Halfter, W, Anterograde tracing of retinal axons in the avian embryo with low molecular weight derivatives of biotin. *Dev Biol*, 1987. 119, 322-335.

[151] Ichijo, H, Differentiation of the chick retinotectal topographic map by remodeling in specificity and refinement in accuracy. *Brain Res Dev Brain Res*, 1999. 117, 199-211.

[152] Baker, RK and Antin, PB, Ephs and ephrins during early stages of chick embryogenesis. *Dev Dyn*, 2003. 228, 128-142.

[153] Schulte, D and Cepko, CL, Two homeobox genes define the domain of epha3 expression in the developing chick retina. *Development*, 2000. 127, 5033-5045.

[154] Cheng, HJ, Nakamoto, M, Bergemann, AD and Flanagan, JG, Complementary gradients in expression and binding of elf-1 and mek4 in development of the topographic retinotectal projection map. *Cell*, 1995. 82, 371-381.

[155] Yamagata, M, Mai, A, Pollerberg, GE and Noda, M, Regulatory interrelations among topographic molecules cbf1, cbf2 and epha3 in the developing chick retina. *Dev Growth Differ*, 1999. 41, 575-587.

[156] Connor, RJ, Menzel, P and Pasquale, EB, Expression and tyrosine phosphorylation of eph receptors suggest multiple mechanisms in patterning of the visual system. *Dev Biol*, 1998. 193, 21-35.

[157] Holash, JA and Pasquale, EB, Polarized expression of the receptor protein tyrosine kinase cek5 in the developing avian visual system. *Dev Biol*, 1995. 172, 683-693.

[158] Soans, C, Holash, JA, Pavlova, Y and Pasquale, EB, Developmental expression and distinctive tyrosine phosphorylation of the eph-related receptor tyrosine kinase cek9. *J Cell Biol*, 1996. 135, 781-795.

[159] Mey, J and Thanos, S, Development of the visual system of the chick--a review. *J Hirnforsch*, 1992. 33, 673-702.

[160] Rager, U, Rager, G and Frei, B, Central retinal area is not the site where ganglion cells are generated first. *J Comp Neurol*, 1993. 334, 529-544.

[161] Sefton, M, Araujo, M and Nieto, MA, Novel expression gradients of eph-like receptor tyrosine kinases in the developing chick retina. *Dev Biol*, 1997. 188, 363-368.

[162] Sen, J, Harpavat, S, Peters, MA and Cepko, CL, Retinoic acid regulates the expression of dorsoventral topographic guidance molecules in the chick retina. *Development*, 2005. 132, 5147-5159.

[163] Braisted, JE, McLaughlin, T, Wang, HU, Friedman, GC, Anderson, DJ, and O'Leary, DD, Graded and lamina-specific distributions of ligands of ephb receptor tyrosine kinases in the developing retinotectal system. *Dev Biol*, 1997. 191, 14-28.

[164] Kalo, MS, Yu, HH and Pasquale, EB, In vivo tyrosine phosphorylation sites of activated ephrin-b1 and ephb2 from neural tissue. *J Biol Chem*, 2001. 276, 38940-38948.

[165] Dutting, D, Handwerker, C and Drescher, U, Topographic targeting and pathfinding errors of retinal axons following overexpression of ephrina ligands on retinal ganglion cell axons. *Dev Biol*, 1999. 216, 297-311.

[166] Peters, MA and Cepko, CL, The dorsal-ventral axis of the neural retina is divided into multiple domains of restricted gene expression which exhibit features of lineage compartments. *Dev Biol*, 2002. 251, 59-73.

[167] Drescher, U, Kremoser, C, Handwerker, C, Loschinger, J, Noda, M, and Bonhoeffer, F, In vitro guidance of retinal ganglion cell axons by rags, a 25 kda tectal protein related to ligands for eph receptor tyrosine kinases. *Cell*, 1995. 82, 359-370.

[168] Monschau, B, Kremoser, C, Ohta, K, Tanaka, H, Kaneko, T, Yamada, T, ... Drescher, U, Shared and distinct functions of rags and elf-1 in guiding retinal axons. *EMBO J*, 1997. 16, 1258-1267.

[169] Marin, O, Blanco, MJ and Nieto, MA, Differential expression of eph receptors and ephrins correlates with the formation of topographic projections in primary and secondary visual circuits of the embryonic chick forebrain. *Dev Biol*, 2001. 234, 289-303.

[170] Hindges, R, McLaughlin, T, Genoud, N, Henkemeyer, M and O'Leary, DD, Ephb forward signaling controls directional branch extension and

arborization required for dorsal-ventral retinotopic mapping. *Neuron*, 2002. 35, 475-487.

[171] Holash, JA, Soans, C, Chong, LD, Shao, H, Dixit, VM, and Pasquale, EB, Reciprocal expression of the eph receptor cek5 and its ligand(s) in the early retina. *Dev Biol*, 1997. 182, 256-269.

[172] Graw, J, Eye development. *Curr Top Dev Biol*, 2010. 90, 343-386.

[173] Farah, MH and Easter, SS, Jr., Cell birth and death in the mouse retinal ganglion cell layer. *J Comp Neurol*, 2005. 489, 120-134.

[174] Gan, L, Xiang, M, Zhou, L, Wagner, DS, Klein, WH, and Nathans, J, Pou domain factor brn-3b is required for the development of a large set of retinal ganglion cells. *Proc Natl Acad Sci U S A*, 1996. 93, 3920-3925.

[175] Colello, RJ and Guillery, RW, The early development of retinal ganglion cells with uncrossed axons in the mouse: Retinal position and axonal course. *Development*, 1990. 108, 515-523.

[176] Godement, P, Salaun, J and Imbert, M, Prenatal and postnatal development of retinogeniculate and retinocollicular projections in the mouse. *J Comp Neurol*, 1984. 230, 552-575.

[177] Brown, A, Yates, PA, Burrola, P, Ortuno, D, Vaidya, A, Jessell, TM, ... Lemke, G, Topographic mapping from the retina to the midbrain is controlled by relative but not absolute levels of epha receptor signaling. *Cell*, 2000. 102, 77-88.

[178] Feldheim, DA, Nakamoto, M, Osterfield, M, Gale, NW, DeChiara, TM, Rohatgi, R, ... Flanagan, JG, Loss-of-function analysis of epha receptors in retinotectal mapping. *J Neurosci*, 2004. 24, 2542-2550.

[179] Cooper, MA, Crockett, DP, Nowakowski, RS, Gale, NW and Zhou, R, Distribution of epha5 receptor protein in the developing and adult mouse nervous system. *J Comp Neurol*, 2009. 514, 310-328.

[180] Carreres, MI, Escalante, A, Murillo, B, Chauvin, G, Gaspar, P, Vegar, C, and Herrera, E, Transcription factor foxd1 is required for the specification of the temporal retina in mammals. *J Neurosci*, 2011. 31, 5673-5681.

[181] Diaz, E, Yang, YH, Ferreira, T, Loh, KC, Okazaki, Y, Hayashizaki, Y, ... Ngai, J, Analysis of gene expression in the developing mouse retina. *Proc Natl Acad Sci U S A*, 2003. 100, 5491-5496.

[182] Bovolenta, P and Mason, C, Growth cone morphology varies with position in the developing mouse visual pathway from retina to first targets. *J Neurosci*, 1987. 7, 1447-1460.

[183] Godement, P, Vanselow, J, Thanos, S and Bonhoeffer, F, A study in developing visual systems with a new method of staining neurones and their processes in fixed tissue. *Development*, 1987. 101, 697-713.

[184] Feldheim, DA, Vanderhaeghen, P, Hansen, MJ, Frisen, J, Lu, Q, Barbacid, M, and Flanagan, JG, Topographic guidance labels in a sensory projection to the forebrain. *Neuron*, 1998. 21, 1303-1313.

[185] Feldheim, DA, Kim, YI, Bergemann, AD, Frisen, J, Barbacid, M, and Flanagan, JG, Genetic analysis of ephrin-a2 and ephrin-a5 shows their requirement in multiple aspects of retinocollicular mapping. *Neuron*, 2000. 25, 563-574.

[186] Ellis, J, Liu, Q, Breitman, M, Jenkins, NA, Gilbert, DJ, Copeland, NG, ... et al., Embryo brain kinase: A novel gene of the eph/elk receptor tyrosine kinase family. *Mech Dev*, 1995. 52, 319-341.

[187] Ciossek, T, Monschau, B, Kremoser, C, Loschinger, J, Lang, S, Muller, BK, ... Drescher, U, Eph receptor-ligand interactions are necessary for guidance of retinal ganglion cell axons in vitro. *Eur J Neurosci*, 1998. 10, 1574-1580.

[188] Rodger, J, Lindsey, KA, Leaver, SG, King, CE, Dunlop, SA, and Beazley, LD, Expression of ephrin-a2 in the superior colliculus and epha5 in the retina following optic nerve section in adult rat. *Eur J Neurosci*, 2001. 14, 1929-1936.

[189] Rodgers, ND, Jiao, X and Kiledjian, M, Identifying mrnas bound by rna-binding proteins using affinity purification and differential display. *Methods*, 2002. 26, 115-122.

[190] Reber, M, Burrola, P and Lemke, G, A relative signalling model for the formation of a topographic neural map. *Nature*, 2004. 431, 847-853.

[191] Petros, TJ, Williams, SE and Mason, CA, Temporal regulation of epha4 in astroglia during murine retinal and optic nerve development. *Mol Cell Neurosci*, 2006. 32, 49-66.

[192] Williams, SE, Mann, F, Erskine, L, Sakurai, T, Wei, S, Rossi, DJ, ... Henkemeyer, M, Ephrin-b2 and ephb1 mediate retinal axon divergence at the optic chiasm. *Neuron*, 2003. 39, 919-935.

[193] Birgbauer, E, Cowan, CA, Sretavan, DW and Henkemeyer, M, Kinase independent function of ephb receptors in retinal axon pathfinding to the optic disc from dorsal but not ventral retina. *Development*, 2000. 127, 1231-1241.

[194] Marcus, RC, Gale, NW, Morrison, ME, Mason, CA and Yancopoulos, GD, Eph family receptors and their ligands distribute in opposing gradients in the developing mouse retina. *Dev Biol*, 1996. 180, 786-789.

[195] Diez-Roux, G, Banfi, S, Sultan, M, Geffers, L, Anand, S, Rozado, D, ... Ballabio, A, A high-resolution anatomical atlas of the transcriptome in the mouse embryo. *PLoS Biol*, 2011. 9, e1000582.

[196] Drager, UC, Birth dates of retinal ganglion cells giving rise to the crossed and uncrossed optic projections in the mouse. *Proc R Soc Lond B Biol Sci*, 1985. 224, 57-77.

[197] Pfeiffenberger, C, Cutforth, T, Woods, G, Yamada, J, Renteria, RC, Copenhagen, DR, ... Feldheim, DA, Ephrin-as and neural activity are required for eye-specific patterning during retinogeniculate mapping. *Nat Neurosci*, 2005. 8, 1022-1027.

[198] Cheng, HJ and Flanagan, JG, Identification and cloning of elf-1, a developmentally expressed ligand for the mek4 and sek receptor tyrosine kinases. *Cell*, 1994. 79, 157-168.

[199] Frisen, J, Yates, PA, McLaughlin, T, Friedman, GC, O'Leary, DD, and Barbacid, M, Ephrin-a5 (al-1/rags) is essential for proper retinal axon guidance and topographic mapping in the mammalian visual system. *Neuron*, 1998. 20, 235-243.

[200] Knoll, B, Isenmann, S, Kilic, E, Walkenhorst, J, Engel, S, Wehinger, J, ... Drescher, U, Graded expression patterns of ephrin-as in the superior colliculus after lesion of the adult mouse optic nerve. *Mech Dev*, 2001. 106, 119-127.

[201] Greferath, U, Canty, AJ, Messenger, J and Murphy, M, Developmental expression of epha4-tyrosine kinase receptor in the mouse brain and spinal cord. *Mech Dev*, 2002. 119 Suppl 1, S231-238.

[202] Jackson, CA and Hickey, TL, Use of ferrets in studies of the visual system. *Lab Anim Sci*, 1985. 35, 211-215.

[203] Greiner, JV and Weidman, TA, Histogenesis of the ferret retina. *Exp Eye Res*, 1981. 33, 315-332.

[204] Reese, BE, Thompson, WF and Peduzzi, JD, Birthdates of neurons in the retinal ganglion cell layer of the ferret. *J Comp Neurol*, 1994. 341, 464-475.

[205] Johnson, JK and Casagrande, VA, Prenatal development of axon outgrowth and connectivity in the ferret visual system. *Vis Neurosci*, 1993. 10, 117-130.

[206] Huberman, AD, Murray, KD, Warland, DK, Feldheim, DA and Chapman, B, Ephrin-as mediate targeting of eye-specific projections to the lateral geniculate nucleus. *Nat Neurosci*, 2005. 8, 1013-1021.

[207] Jeffery, G, Retinotopic order appears before ocular separation in developing visual pathways. *Nature*, 1985. 313, 575-576.

[208] Linden, DC, Guillery, RW and Cucchiaro, J, The dorsal lateral geniculate nucleus of the normal ferret and its postnatal development. *J Comp Neurol*, 1981. 203, 189-211.

[209] Zahs, KR and Stryker, MP, The projection of the visual field onto the lateral geniculate nucleus of the ferret. *J Comp Neurol*, 1985. 241, 210-224.

[210] Jeffery, G, Shifting retinal maps in the development of the lateral geniculate nucleus. *Brain Res Dev Brain Res*, 1989. 46, 187-196.

[211] Zhang, J, Rubin, RM and Rao, NA, Anatomy and embryology of the optic nerve. *Duanes Ophthalmology*, 2006. Lippencott, Williams and Wilkens, Chapter 27.

[212] Mann, I, The development of the human eye. *The University Press*, 1928.

[213] O'Brien, KM, Schulte, D and Hendrickson, AE, Expression of photoreceptor-associated molecules during human fetal eye development. *Mol Vis*, 2003. 9, 401-409.

[214] La Vail, MM, Rapaport, DH and Rakic, P, Cytogenesis in the monkey retina. *J Comp Neurol*, 1991. 309, 86-114.

[215] Lambot, MA, Depasse, F, Noel, JC and Vanderhaeghen, P, Mapping labels in the human developing visual system and the evolution of binocular vision. *J Neurosci*, 2005. 25, 7232-7237.

[216] Kozulin, P, Natoli, R, Madigan, MC, O'Brien, KM and Provis, JM, Gradients of eph-a6 expression in primate retina suggest roles in both vascular and axon guidance. *Mol Vis*, 2009. 15, 2649-2662.

[217] Kozulin, P, Natoli, R, O'Brien, KM, Madigan, MC and Provis, JM, Differential expression of anti-angiogenic factors and guidance genes in the developing macula. *Mol Vis*, 2009. 15, 45-59.

[218] Kozulin, P and Provis, JM, Differential gene expression in the developing human macula: Microarray analysis using rare tissue samples. *J Ocul Biol Dis Infor*, 2009. 2, 176-189.

[219] Hevner, RF, Development of connections in the human visual system during fetal mid-gestation: A dii-tracing study. *J Neuropathol Exp Neurol*, 2000. 59, 385-392.

[220] Bao, ZZ, Intraretinal projection of retinal ganglion cell axons as a model system for studying axon navigation. *Brain Res*, 2008. 1192, 165-177.

[221] Brittis, PA and Silver, J, Multiple factors govern intraretinal axon guidance: A time-lapse study. *Mol Cell Neurosci*, 1995. 6, 413-432.

[222] Becker, CG and Becker, T, Repellent guidance of regenerating optic axons by chondroitin sulfate glycosaminoglycans in zebrafish. *J Neurosci*, 2002. 22, 842-853.

[223] Reese, BE, Development of the retina and optic pathway. *Vision Res*, 2011. 51, 613-632.

[224] Petros, TJ, Rebsam, A and Mason, CA, Retinal axon growth at the optic chiasm: To cross or not to cross. *Annu Rev Neurosci*, 2008. 31, 295-315.

[225] Meissirel, C, Wikler, KC, Chalupa, LM and Rakic, P, Early divergence of magnocellular and parvocellular functional subsystems in the embryonic primate visual system. *Proc Natl Acad Sci U S A*, 1997. 94, 5900-5905.

[226] Wang, LC, Rachel, RA, Marcus, RC and Mason, CA, Chemosuppression of retinal axon growth by the mouse optic chiasm. *Neuron*, 1996. 17, 849-862.

[227] Petros, TJ, Shrestha, BR and Mason, C, Specificity and sufficiency of ephb1 in driving the ipsilateral retinal projection. *J Neurosci*, 2009. 29, 3463-3474.

[228] Garcia-Frigola, C, Carreres, MI, Vegar, C, Mason, C and Herrera, E, Zic2 promotes axonal divergence at the optic chiasm midline by ephb1-dependent and -independent mechanisms. *Development*, 2008. 135, 1833-1841.

[229] Burrill, JD and Easter, SS, Jr., Development of the retinofugal projections in the embryonic and larval zebrafish (brachydanio rerio). *J Comp Neurol*, 1994. 346, 583-600.

[230] Nakagawa, S, Brennan, C, Johnson, KG, Shewan, D, Harris, WA, and Holt, CE, Ephrin-b regulates the ipsilateral routing of retinal axons at the optic chiasm. *Neuron*, 2000. 25, 599-610.

[231] Chenaux, G and Henkemeyer, M, Forward signaling by ephb1/ephb2 interacting with ephrin-b ligands at the optic chiasm is required to form the ipsilateral projection. *Eur J Neurosci*, 2011. 34, 1620-1633.

[232] Becker, N, Seitanidou, T, Murphy, P, Mattei, MG, Topilko, P, Nieto, MA, ... Gilardi-Hebenstreit, P, Several receptor tyrosine kinase genes of the eph family are segmentally expressed in the developing hindbrain. *Mech Dev*, 1994. 47, 3-17.

[233] Walkenhorst, J, Dutting, D, Handwerker, C, Huai, J, Tanaka, H, and Drescher, U, The epha4 receptor tyrosine kinase is necessary for the guidance of nasal retinal ganglion cell axons in vitro. *Mol Cell Neurosci*, 2000. 16, 365-375.

[234] Marcus, RC, Matthews, GA, Gale, NW, Yancopoulos, GD and Mason, CA, Axon guidance in the mouse optic chiasm: Retinal neurite inhibition by ephrin "a"-expressing hypothalamic cells in vitro. *Dev Biol*, 2000. 221, 132-147.

[235] Knoll, B and Drescher, U, Ephrin-as as receptors in topographic projections. *Trends Neurosci*, 2002. 25, 145-149.

[236] Cohen-Cory, S and Lom, B, Neurotrophic regulation of retinal ganglion cell synaptic connectivity: From axons and dendrites to synapses. *Int J Dev Biol*, 2004. 48, 947-956.

[237] Suzuki, A, Nomura, S, Morii, E, Fukuda, Y and Kosaka, J, Localization of mrnas for trkb isoforms and p75 in rat retinal ganglion cells. *J Neurosci Res*, 1998. 54, 27-37.

[238] Ugolini, G, Cremisi, F and Maffei, L, Trka, trkb and p75 mrna expression is developmentally regulated in the rat retina. *Brain Res*, 1995. 704, 121-124.

[239] Lebrun-Julien, F and Di Polo, A, Molecular and cell-based approaches for neuroprotection in glaucoma. *Optom Vis Sci*, 2008. 85, 417-424.

[240] Johnson, TV, Bull, ND and Martin, KR, Neurotrophic factor delivery as a protective treatment for glaucoma. *Exp Eye Res*, 2011. 93, 196-203.

[241] Weber, AJ, Harman, CD and Viswanathan, S, Effects of optic nerve injury, glaucoma, and neuroprotection on the survival, structure, and function of ganglion cells in the mammalian retina. *J Physiol*, 2008. 586, 4393-4400.

[242] Isenmann, S, Kretz, A and Cellerino, A, Molecular determinants of retinal ganglion cell development, survival, and regeneration. *Prog Retin Eye Res*, 2003. 22, 483-543.

[243] Ruthazer, ES and Cline, HT, Insights into activity-dependent map formation from the retinotectal system: A middle-of-the-brain perspective. *J Neurobiol*, 2004. 59, 134-146.

[244] Goodhill, GJ and Richards, LJ, Retinotectal maps: Molecules, models and misplaced data. *Trends Neurosci*, 1999. 22, 529-534.

[245] Simpson, HD, Mortimer, D and Goodhill, GJ, Theoretical models of neural circuit development. *Curr Top Dev Biol*, 2009. 87, 1-51.

[246] Yates, PA, Holub, AD, McLaughlin, T, Sejnowski, TJ and O'Leary, DD, Computational modeling of retinotopic map development to define contributions of epha-ephrina gradients, axon-axon interactions, and patterned activity. *J Neurobiol*, 2004. 59, 95-113.

[247] Tsigankov, DN and Koulakov, AA, A unifying model for activity-dependent and activity-independent mechanisms predicts complete

structure of topographic maps in ephrin-a deficient mice. *J Comput Neurosci*, 2006. 21, 101-114.

[248] Godfrey, KB, Eglen, SJ and Swindale, NV, A multi-component model of the developing retinocollicular pathway incorporating axonal and synaptic growth. *PLoS Comput Biol*, 2009. 5, e1000600.

[249] Gebhardt, C, Bastmeyer, M and Weth, F, Balancing of ephrin/eph forward and reverse signaling as the driving force of adaptive topographic mapping. *Development*, 2012. 139, 335-345.

[250] Grimbert, F and Cang, J, New model of retinocollicular mapping predicts the mechanisms of axonal competition and explains the role of reverse molecular signaling during development. *J Neurosci*, 2012. 32, 9755-9768.

[251] Meyer, JS, Howden, SE, Wallace, KA, Verhoeven, AD, Wright, LS, Capowski, EE, ... Gamm, DM, Optic vesicle-like structures derived from human pluripotent stem cells facilitate a customized approach to retinal disease treatment. *Stem Cells*, 2011. 29, 1206-1218.

[252] Mellough, CB, Sernagor, E, Moreno-Gimeno, I, Steel, DH and Lako, M, Efficient stage-specific differentiation of human pluripotent stem cells toward retinal photoreceptor cells. *Stem Cells*, 2012. 30, 673-686.

[253] Ramsden, CM, Powner, MB, Carr, AJ, Smart, MJ, da Cruz, L, and Coffey, PJ, Stem cells in retinal regeneration: Past, present and future. *Development*, 2013. 140, 2576-2585.

[254] Osakada, F, Hirami, Y and Takahashi, M, Stem cell biology and cell transplantation therapy in the retina. *Biotechnol Genet Eng Rev*, 2010. 26, 297-334.

[255] Zupanc, GK and Sirbulescu, RF, Adult neurogenesis and neuronal regeneration in the central nervous system of teleost fish. *Eur J Neurosci*, 2011. 34, 917-929.

[256] Otteson, DC and Hitchcock, PF, Stem cells in the teleost retina: Persistent neurogenesis and injury-induced regeneration. *Vision Res*, 2003. 43, 927-936.

[257] Matsukawa, T, Arai, K, Koriyama, Y, Liu, Z and Kato, S, Axonal regeneration of fish optic nerve after injury. *Biol Pharm Bull*, 2004. 27, 445-451.

[258] Hitchcock, P, Ochocinska, M, Sieh, A and Otteson, D, Persistent and injury-induced neurogenesis in the vertebrate retina. *Prog Retin Eye Res*, 2004. 23, 183-194.

[259] Raymond, PA and Hitchcock, PF, How the neural retina regenerates. *Results Probl Cell Differ*, 2000. 31, 197-218.

[260] Rodger, J, Symonds, AC, Springbett, J, Shen, WY, Bartlett, CA, Rakoczy, PE, ... Dunlop, SA, Eph/ephrin expression in the adult rat visual system following localized retinal lesions: Localized and transneuronal up-regulation in the retina and superior colliculus. *Eur J Neurosci*, 2005. 22, 1840-1852.

[261] Symonds, AC, King, CE, Bartlett, CA, Sauve, Y, Lund, RD, Beazley, LD, ... Rodger, J, Epha5 and ephrin-a2 expression during optic nerve regeneration: A 'two-edged sword'. *Eur J Neurosci*, 2007. 25, 744-752.

[262] Munemasa, Y and Kitaoka, Y, Molecular mechanisms of retinal ganglion cell degeneration in glaucoma and future prospects for cell body and axonal protection. *Front Cell Neurosci*, 2012. 6, 60.

[263] Colak, D, Morales, J, Bosley, TM, Al-Bakheet, A, AlYounes, B, Kaya, N, and Abu-Amero, KK, Genome-wide expression profiling of patients with primary open angle glaucoma. *Invest Ophthalmol Vis Sci*, 2012. 53, 5899-5904.

[264] Guo, Y, Johnson, EC, Cepurna, WO, Dyck, JA, Doser, T, and Morrison, JC, Early gene expression changes in the retinal ganglion cell layer of a rat glaucoma model. *Invest Ophthalmol Vis Sci*, 2011. 52, 1460-1473.

[265] Steele, MR, Inman, DM, Calkins, DJ, Horner, PJ and Vetter, ML, Microarray analysis of retinal gene expression in the dba/2j model of glaucoma. *Invest Ophthalmol Vis Sci*, 2006. 47, 977-985.

[266] Schmidt, J, Agapova, OA, Yang, P, Kaufman, PL and Hernandez, MR, Expression of ephrinb1 and its receptor in glaucomatous optic neuropathy. *Br J Ophthalmol*, 2007.

[267] Cui, X, Xu, N, Liao, W, Xu, J, Ge, C, Ye, J, ... He, X, Gene expression profile determination in rat retinal tissue after ocular hypertension through oligo microarray. *Ophthalmic Res*, 2011. 45, 57-64.

[268] Panagis, L, Zhao, X, Ge, Y, Ren, L, Mittag, TW, and Danias, J, Gene expression changes in areas of focal loss of retinal ganglion cells in the retina of dba/2j mice. *Invest Ophthalmol Vis Sci*, 2010. 51, 2024-2034.

[269] Guo, L, Salt, TE, Maass, A, Luong, V, Moss, SE, Fitzke, FW, and Cordeiro, MF, Assessment of neuroprotective effects of glutamate modulation on glaucoma-related retinal ganglion cell apoptosis in vivo. *Invest Ophthalmol Vis Sci*, 2006. 47, 626-633.

[270] Miyahara, T, Kikuchi, T, Akimoto, M, Kurokawa, T, Shibuki, H, and Yoshimura, N, Gene microarray analysis of experimental glaucomatous retina from cynomologous monkey. *Invest Ophthalmol Vis Sci*, 2003. 44, 4347-4356.

[271] Hernandez, MR, Agapova, OA, Yang, P, Salvador-Silva, M, Ricard, CS, and Aoi, S, Differential gene expression in astrocytes from human normal and glaucomatous optic nerve head analyzed by cdna microarray. *Glia*, 2002. 38, 45-64.

[272] Du, J, Tran, T, Fu, C and Sretavan, DW, Upregulation of ephb2 and ephrin-b2 at the optic nerve head of dba/2j glaucomatous mice coincides with axon loss. *Invest Ophthalmol Vis Sci*, 2007. 48, 5567-5581.

[273] Fu, CT, Tran, T and Sretavan, D, Axonal/glial upregulation of ephb/ephrin-b signaling in mouse experimental ocular hypertension. *Invest Ophthalmol Vis Sci*, 2010. 51, 991-1001.

[274] Fu, CT and Sretavan, D, Involvement of ephb/ephrin-b signaling in axonal survival in mouse experimental glaucoma. *Invest Ophthalmol Vis Sci*, 2012. 53, 76-84.

[275] Arvanitis, DN and Davy, A, Regulation and misregulation of eph/ephrin expression. *Cell Adh Migr*, 2012. 6, 131-137.

[276] Hatini, V, Tao, W and Lai, E, Expression of winged helix genes, bf-1 and bf-2, define adjacent domains within the developing forebrain and retina. *J Neurobiol*, 1994. 25, 1293-1309.

[277] Takahashi, H, Shintani, T, Sakuta, H and Noda, M, Cbf1 controls the retinotectal topographical map along the anteroposterior axis through multiple mechanisms. *Development*, 2003. 130, 5203-5215.

[278] Takahashi, H, Sakuta, H, Shintani, T and Noda, M, Functional mode of foxd1/cbf2 for the establishment of temporal retinal specificity in the developing chick retina. *Dev Biol*, 2009. 331, 300-310.

[279] Yuasa, J, Hirano, S, Yamagata, M and Noda, M, Visual projection map specified by topographic expression of transcription factors in the retina. *Nature*, 1996. 382, 632-635.

[280] Wang, W, Lo, P, Frasch, M and Lufkin, T, Hmx: An evolutionary conserved homeobox gene family expressed in the developing nervous system in mice and drosophila. *Mech Dev*, 2000. 99, 123-137.

[281] Boisset, G and Schorderet, DF, Zebrafish hmx1 promotes retinogenesis. *Exp Eye Res*, 2012. 105, 34-42.

[282] Munroe, RJ, Prabhu, V, Acland, GM, Johnson, KR, Harris, BS, O'Brien, TP, ... Schimenti, JC, Mouse h6 homeobox 1 (hmx1) mutations cause cranial abnormalities and reduced body mass. *BMC Dev Biol*, 2009. 9, 27.

[283] Vaclavik, V, Schorderet, DF, Borruat, FX and Munier, FL, Retinal dystrophy in the oculo-auricular syndrome due to hmx1 mutation. *Ophthalmic Genet*, 2011. 32, 114-117.

[284] Schorderet, DF, Nichini, O, Boisset, G, Polok, B, Tiab, L, Mayeur, H, ... Munier, FL, Mutation in the human homeobox gene nkx5-3 causes an oculo-auricular syndrome. *Am J Hum Genet*, 2008. 82, 1178-1184.

[285] Herrera, E, Brown, L, Aruga, J, Rachel, RA, Dolen, G, Mikoshiba, K, ... Mason, CA, Zic2 patterns binocular vision by specifying the uncrossed retinal projection. *Cell*, 2003. 114, 545-557.

[286] Pak, W, Hindges, R, Lim, YS, Pfaff, SL and O'Leary, DD, Magnitude of binocular vision controlled by islet-2 repression of a genetic program that specifies laterality of retinal axon pathfinding. *Cell*, 2004. 119, 567-578.

[287] Lee, R, Petros, TJ and Mason, CA, Zic2 regulates retinal ganglion cell axon avoidance of ephrinb2 through inducing expression of the guidance receptor ephb1. *J Neurosci*, 2008. 28, 5910-5919.

[288] Tam, PP, Loebel, DA and Tanaka, SS, Building the mouse gastrula: Signals, asymmetry and lineages. *Curr Opin Genet Dev*, 2006. 16, 419-425.

[289] Schmitt, AM, Shi, J, Wolf, AM, Lu, CC, King, LA, and Zou, Y, Wnt-ryk signalling mediates medial-lateral retinotectal topographic mapping. *Nature*, 2006. 439, 31-37.

[290] de Iongh, RU, Abud, HE and Hime, GR, Wnt/frizzled signaling in eye development and disease. *Front Biosci*, 2006. 11, 2442-2464.

[291] Van Raay, TJ and Vetter, ML, Wnt/frizzled signaling during vertebrate retinal development. *Dev Neurosci*, 2004. 26, 352-358.

[292] Chien, AJ, Conrad, WH and Moon, RT, A wnt survival guide: From flies to human disease. *J Invest Dermatol*, 2009. 129, 1614-1627.

[293] Gao, C and Chen, YG, Dishevelled: The hub of wnt signaling. *Cell Signal*, 2010. 22, 717-727.

[294] Tanaka, M, Kamo, T, Ota, S and Sugimura, H, Association of dishevelled with eph tyrosine kinase receptor and ephrin mediates cell repulsion. *EMBO J*, 2003. 22, 847-858.

[295] Meissner, A, Mikkelsen, TS, Gu, H, Wernig, M, Hanna, J, Sivachenko, A, ... Lander, ES, Genome-scale DNA methylation maps of pluripotent and differentiated cells. *Nature*, 2008. 454, 766-770.

[296] Bird, A, DNA methylation patterns and epigenetic memory. *Genes Dev*, 2002. 16, 6-21.

[297] Dawson, DW, Hong, JS, Shen, RR, French, SW, Troke, JJ, Wu, YZ, ... Teitell, MA, Global DNA methylation profiling reveals silencing of a secreted form of epha7 in mouse and human germinal center b-cell lymphomas. *Oncogene*, 2007. 26, 4243-4252.

[298] Dottori, M, Down, M, Huttmann, A, Fitzpatrick, DR and Boyd, AW, Cloning and characterization of epha3 (hek) gene promoter: DNA methylation regulates expression in hematopoietic tumor cells. *Blood*, 1999. 94, 2477-2486.

[299] Fu, DY, Wang, ZM, Wang, BL, Chen, L, Yang, WT, Shen, ZZ, ... Shao, ZM, Frequent epigenetic inactivation of the receptor tyrosine kinase epha5 by promoter methylation in human breast cancer. *Hum Pathol*, 2010. 41, 48-58.

[300] Kuang, SQ, Bai, H, Fang, ZH, Lopez, G, Yang, H, Tong, W, ... Garcia-Manero, G, Aberrant DNA methylation and epigenetic inactivation of eph receptor tyrosine kinases and ephrin ligands in acute lymphoblastic leukemia. *Blood*, 2010. 115, 2412-2419.

[301] Wang, J, Kataoka, H, Suzuki, M, Sato, N, Nakamura, R, Tao, H, ... Sugimura, H, Downregulation of epha7 by hypermethylation in colorectal cancer. *Oncogene*, 2005. 24, 5637-5647.

[302] Wang, J, Li, G, Ma, H, Bao, Y, Wang, X, Zhou, H, ... Zhou, X, Differential expression of epha7 receptor tyrosine kinase in gastric carcinoma. *Hum Pathol*, 2007. 38, 1649-1656.

[303] Wang, JD, Dong, YC, Sheng, Z, Ma, HH, Li, GL, Wang, XL, ... Zhou, XJ, Loss of expression of ephb1 protein in gastric carcinoma associated with invasion and metastasis. *Oncology*, 2007. 73, 238-245.

[304] Kalinski, T, Ropke, A, Sel, S, Kouznetsova, I, Ropke, M, and Roessner, A, Down-regulation of ephrin-a5, a gene product of normal cartilage, in chondrosarcoma. *Hum Pathol*, 2009. 40, 1679-1685.

[305] Merlos-Suarez, A and Batlle, E, Eph-ephrin signalling in adult tissues and cancer. *Curr Opin Cell Biol*, 2008. 20, 194-200.

[306] Petkova, TD, Seigel, GM and Otteson, DC, A role for DNA methylation in regulation of epha5 receptor expression in the mouse retina. *Vision Res*, 2011. 51, 260-268.

[307] Moore, DL, Blackmore, MG, Hu, Y, Kaestner, KH, Bixby, JL, Lemmon, VP, and Goldberg, JL, Klf family members regulate intrinsic axon regeneration ability. *Science*, 2009. 326, 298-301.

[308] Goodhill, GJ and Xu, J, The development of retinotectal maps: A review of models based on molecular gradients. *Network*, 2005. 16, 5-34.

[309] Tsigankov, D and Koulakov, AA, Sperry versus hebb: Topographic mapping in isl2/epha3 mutant mice. *BMC Neurosci*, 2010. 11, 155.

[310] Sterratt, DC and Hjorth, JJ, Retinocollicular mapping explained? *Vis Neurosci*, 2013. 30, 125-128.

[311] O'Leary, DD and McLaughlin, T, Mechanisms of retinotopic map development: Ephs, ephrins, and spontaneous correlated retinal activity. *Prog Brain Res*, 2005. 147, 43-65.

In: Ganglion Cells
Editor: Liora G. Vlastimil

ISBN: 978-1-63117-432-2

Chapter 2

NONVISUAL GANGLION CELL SUBTYPE: WHICH KIND OF CELLS ARE THEY? AND WHERE DO THEY COME FROM?

Javier Vicente, Pedro de la Villa and Francisco Germain*

Department of Biology of Systems, School of Medicine, University of Alcalá, Campus Universitario, Alcalá de Henares, Madrid, Spain

ABSTRACT

Mammalian photoreception requires the presence of photosensitive cells in the retina. This process takes place thanks to a protein (opsin), which contains a cromophore. Rods and cones allow mammals, and other multiple species, to see the world around them. Rods and cones were thought to be the only photoreceptors until the last decades. The discovery of a new opsin (melanopsin) inside other retinal cells has finished with the traditional exclusivity of rods and cones as photosensitive cells. In mammals, these cells are localized in the Ganglion Cell Layer. There is a ganglion cell type that contains this photopigment, the melanopsin ganglion cells, commonly known as ipRGCs (intrinsically photosensitive retinal ganglion cells). These cells appear to have a key role in regulating certain aspects of the visual system not related to image formation, as well as various physiological

* Corresponding author: Email: francisco.germain@uah.es.

functions fundamental for the organism: Melanopsin is an important regulator of the circadian clock.

Earlier studies showed how blind individuals with degenerated rod and cone photoreceptors still maintained photoentrainment and the pupillary light reflex. The presence of another photoreceptor was obvious. Melanopsin-containing cells were found in mouse and human retinal ganglion cells, but other animals had amacrine and horizontal cells that also expressed melanopsin. Melanopsin ganglion cells were regarded as the new type of photoreceptor. However, recent studies indicate that ipRGCs are composed of different subtypes. The relation between subtype and function is not always clear. Some of these subtypes share targets in the central nervous system (or even share physiological functions), but they have important morphological differences.

Nowadays, the scientific community accepts the role of the different ipRGCs in non-visual processes, whereas rods and cones are involved in image formation. It is very interesting to study the differences between melanopsin retinal ganglion cells and classical photoreceptors, since their physiological functions are not the only differences. In addition, their molecular requirements and their photochemical properties show a different evolutionary origin. Understanding the evolution and functions of visual and non-visual systems is crucial to understand the functional differences among opsins.

THE AMAZING DISCOVERY

The ability to observe the world around us entails great advantages, in many different ways. We are able to recognize a hazard well in advance because we see it; we can find allies (usually individuals of the same species) because we see them; our foodstuff is composed of a great variety of foods because we see them. Further, thanks to the perception of the world that sight gives us, we can collect information to help us develop feelings, such as trust in others, love and sensations like beauty. However, the mechanism to enjoy this capability is really complex, starting with the structure responsible for receiving, processing and transmitting information to the brain. Not surprisingly, Darwin himself remarked the long and convoluteds journey of evolution to achieve today's degree of complexity [1].

This capacity is provided by visual receptor cells, which perform an amazing job of transforming the energy that comes from light into a type identifiable by the body, electricity. This process is known as phototransduction and is performed by photoreceptor cells, rods and cones, within the CNS structure that supports this function, the retina.

This is possible thanks to the activation of the chromophore (retinal) located inside a protein (opsin). Photoreceptors, by using this photosensitive machinery, enable us to decode the information transmitted by light to reproduce images in the human cerebral cortex.

However, external light is a very important element that not only functions to draw pictures, but also as time reference. This type of factors, which influence us throughout the 24-hour light / dark cycle, are called *zeitgebers* [2]. Light is the most important *zeitgeber* in physiological regulation and animal behavior. Therefore, in addition to having a role in *image formation*, light is considered to exert a great influence on *non-image-forming (NIF)* functions.

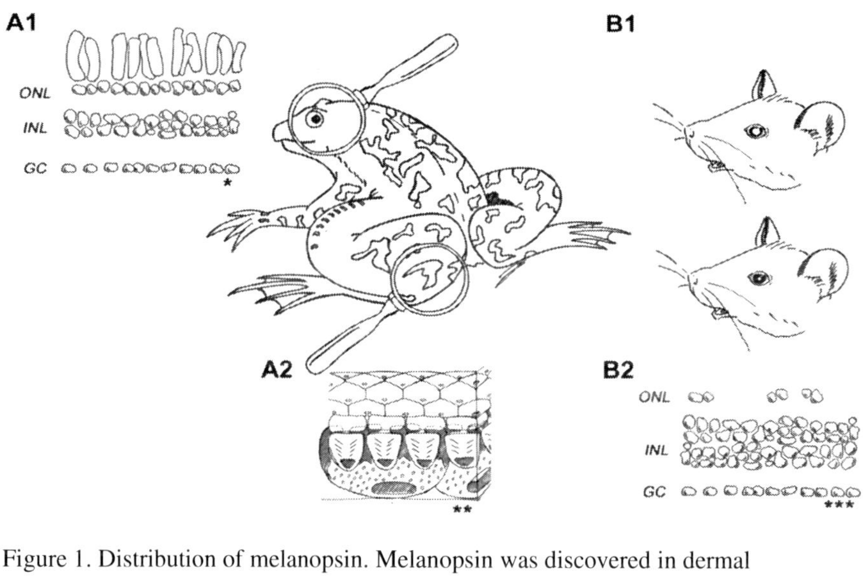

Figure 1. Distribution of melanopsin. Melanopsin was discovered in dermal melanophores of *Xenopus laevis* (**) (**A2**); later, it was also found in the retinal ganglion cell layer (GC), first in amphibians (*) (**A1**), and then in the retina of mammals (***) (**B2**). The pupillary reflex, one of the functions controlled by melanopsin, is also shown **(B1).** Retinal layers: ONL, outer nuclear layer; INL, inner nuclear layer; GC, Ganglion cells.

If it was difficult to understand how these processes, involving classical opsins, rhodopsin and color opsins, were performed, difficulty has increased in recent decades with the discovery of non-classical new opsins [3-5]. Moreover, the finding of these "non-classical" opsins in a ganglion cell subtype increases the number and types of photosensitive cells in the retina.

This ability is due to the presence of a photopigment called melanopsin [6]. It is precisely for that photosensitivity these cells have been called intrinsically photosensitive retinal ganglion cells (ipRGCs) [7].

This discovery has represented and represents a major challenge, as it has forced us to restructure all our knowledge about the functioning of the retina. That is why the axiom that stated the only photoreceptor cells in the retina were the rods and the cones has come to an end.

Melanopsin Discovery: Short History

Previously to the discovery of ipRGCs, some data pointed to the presence of a third photoreceptor. The first clues came from behavioral experiments, molecular and physiological reflex responses. In the early twentieth century, works made with blind mice showed the maintenance of pupillary reflex responses [8]. Decades later, it was observed how the molecular levels of Dopamine and Melatonin showed an increase and a decrease, respectively, conditioned by light, in animals with apparent blindness [9-11]. Also in those years, timing studies showed how circadian rhythms were maintained despite suffering from blindness. This was common to different strains of mouse [12-14]. However, these non-image-forming functions (animals were blind) required illumination of the eye despite the lack of cones and / or rods.

The most convincing evidence of the existence of these new photosensitive cells has been provided in the past 15 years. In 1998, molecular works by Ignacio Provencio showed the presence of a new opsin in dermal melanophores of *Xenopus laevis* [6] (see Figure 1). This opsin was named melanopsin due to its origin, although it had also been found in the brain and the eye of amphibians. In the following years, its location within the mammalian retina was known [15, 16].

These melanopsin ganglion cells were found to be the same light responsive cells recorded by Berson and colleagues [7]. Using the patch-clamp technique, they observed that SCN (suprachiasmatic nucleus)-projecting ganglion cells responded to light after blocking the signals coming from rods and cones. Simultaneously, Hattar and collaborators published a study that showed not only the location of these cells in the retina, but also different ipRGCs arborizations in the INL (inner nuclear layer) [17]. For this purpose, through genetic engineering, a tau-lacZ construct was targeted to the melanopsin gene locus in the mouse. Thereby, the enzyme b-galactosidase was expressed instead of melanopsin and revealed by X-gal (5-bromo-4-chloro-3-

indolyl-β-D-galactopyranoside) staining. This procedure showed a stained ganglion cell population comprising 1-3% of the total population. This *knock in* mouse allowed to clearly see the projections of melanopsin cells to central brain regions, mainly those related to non-visual functions, such as the SCN and the OPN (olivary pretectal nucleus), which regulate circadian rhythms and the pupillary reflex, respectively.

So far, the new photosensitive molecule that drove non-image-forming functions was torn between two possible candidates: melanopsin (already mentioned) and cryptochromes, photopigments sensitive to blue light. Cryptochromes are molecules based on flavin, initially found in invertebrates but also present in the mammalian retina as Cry1 and Cry2 [18].

Finally, the balance was tipped on for melanopsin since rd1 transgenic animals lacking this protein lost circadian synchrony (circadian entrainment) and the pupillary reflex [19, 20]. On the contrary, these functions were not completely abolished in a mouse lacking cryptochromes that suffered retinal degeneration [21].

CLASSIFICATION OF IPRGCS

Earlier this century, suspicions about the presence of photosensitive molecules in mammals other than those of classical photoreceptors (rods and cones) were confirmed. Functional work performed on photosensitive non-cone, no-rod cells began to be supplemented with increasing histological or morphological studies. In those years the research for an effective antibody against melanopsin occupied much of the investigation. Through a good marker / ligand for this protein the researchers attempted to locate and analyze new forms of non-image-forming photoreceptors.

Cloning of opsin in *anourous* led to the identification of homologous mammalian opsins, as in man and mouse [15]. The *Xenopus* melanopsin shares structural similarities with all known opsins, including the seven transmembrane domains that are found in the G protein-coupled receptors (GPCRs). These heptahelical proteins provide transduction between extracellular and intracellular signals in many organisms [22, 23]. As in other known opsins, the supporting part of the chromophore in the photopigment is called melanopsin and is involved in the activation of the cascade by absorbing light at specific wavelengths.

Morphological Classifications

In the retina, target cells for the melanopsin antibody are mainly found in the GCL (ganglion cell layer), although some are found as well in the INL. These cells were anatomically described when the presence of melanopsin in cell bodies, dendrites and proximal axonal segment was observed. Thanks to Hattar's morphological studies, published in 2002, we know that the diameter of these melanopsin-expressing, photosensitive cells exceeds 10 µm, which is similar to type III retinal ganglion cells size [17]. In this paper dendritic arborization was also described, reporting stratification in the outer INL subsheet (OFF sublamina). The dendritic tree extension of melanopsin cells occupies a retinal area 30 times larger than their somas' size. To examine their axonal projections, Hattar and colleagues took advantage of the β-galactosidase enzyme activity, expressed from the tau-lacZ construct. This codes for a fusion protein composed of the enzyme and a signal sequence from tau, which allows β-galactosidase to be transported down the axon.

In heterozygous animals, the tau-lacZ construct was transcribed and translated along with the melanopsin gene, so that b-galactosidase was also expressed in melanopsin cells. Exposure to the enzyme substrate, X-gal, allowed studying more precisely both, the characteristics of the cells in the retina, as well as their way to higher centers. This way, axonal target centers such as the SNC, the pretectum (specifically the OPN), the IGL (intergeniculate leaflet) and the VLG (ventral lateral geniculate) were described. Counting of retinal cells labeled with either X-gal or melanopsin antibody showed a population of around 600-800 cells per retina.

The number of melanopsin retinal ganglion cells seemed very low considering the total number of ganglion cells, 48.000-65.000 [24]. However, later studies raised that value to more than double [25-27]. One reason for this imbalance is the uniqueness of the model used by Hattar in 2002, in which the galactosidase activity was undetectable in half of the melanopsin cells, so that they missed a complete subtype of melanopsin ganglion cells. This cell subtype was termed M2 [28], whereas the one mentioned so far was known as M1. The latter is present both, in the GCL, as well as in displaced ganglion cells in the INL. Both subtypes have morphological differences at the level of their processes, while M1 subtype stratifies at the OFF sublamina of the IPL, M2 subtype has dendrites that remain in the ON sublamina. Also, the cellular staining with anti-melanopsin antibody is different in both subtypes; it is fainter in the M2 subtype. This may denote lower protein expression in this cell type. A second explanation for the low RGC counts found initially could be that the β-galactosidase was fused to a tau sequence that promoted the transport of the protein along the axon. A combination of these two conditions might be the cause of a failure to detect a substantial number of melanopsin cell bodies in the retina [25]. Despite the increase in counts, melanopsin ganglion cells comprise only between 1 and 5% of the total population of ganglion cells [29].

Compared with the characteristics of the M1 subtype, cited above, M2 cells display larger soma and a dendritic tree of greater length and complexity. Further, both subtypes differ in their projections rate to higher centers. In particular, the proportion of each subtype to the two main centers not involved in visual functions, the SCN and the OPN, is different; whereas in the SCN most axons originate from M1 cells (80% M1, 20% M2), in the OPN the ratio is more equal (45% M1, 55% M2) [30]. In addition to the detailed study of the M1 subtype (made by Hattar) and the immunocytochemical descriptions that show dendritic branching of M1 and M2 subtypes in both IPL sublaminas (made by Provencio), other studies have allowed to identify more subtypes that coexist in the retina with the two previous. Thus, a third type was described in the mouse retina, specifically in the pupillary reflex circuit. For this purpose a virus that spread retrogradely, the pseudorabies virus, was used.[31].

Schmidt and collaborators, who showed three different subtypes of melanopsin ganglion cells, supported this diversity. They used an animal model (mouse) in which EGFP (enhanced green fluorescent protein) was expressed under the control of the melanopsin promoter [32]. The third subtype shown in this work is called M3. It exhibits dual stratification of its dendritic tree in both IPL sublaminas (ON and OFF), and represents the 26% of the melanopsin retinal ganglion cell population, as estimated by Schmidt. M2 retinal ganglion cells are similar to M3 in size and dendritic tree complexity [33]. Other groups have corroborated the identification of three different subtypes of melanopsin ganglion cells, although the percentages of each subtype vary according to the authors [31, 34]. However, other groups consider these bi-stratified cells an exception because they believe that the new counts appear just occasionally [27, 35]. In primate retina only the first two subtypes (M1 and M2) of melanopsin ganglion cells have been described [36]. The three subtypes were morphologically identified by observing the intrinsic fluorescence of melanopsin-containing cells, through the use of antibodies against the opsin amino and carboxyl ends, and also by using transgenic mice carrying reporter genes.

Functional Classifications

The existence of these subtypes was also corroborated by electrophysiological analysis. Intrinsic light responses are larger and exhibit greater sensitivity in M1 than in M2 melanopsin ganglion cells. The reason why M2 cells are 10 times less sensitive than M1 is, probably, because they have lower levels of melanopsin. Also the membrane potential in darkness varies for both subtypes. It is more positive in M1 than in M2 cells (M1 is more depolarized and M2 more hyperpolarized). Additionally, electrical activity of the M1 subtype has a lower frequency than the M2 [37]. However, in the case of M3 cells, electrophysiological characteristics are similar to those of M2 subtype [38]. Other functional works, without morphological support, had already determined the possible existence of more than one type of melanopsin-containing cells [39, 40]. These studies have allowed us to define this cell group as a class.

Another kind of classification is based on the expression of one or both of the two melanopsin existing isoforms. A paper has been recently published in which the relationship between morphological subtypes and the expression of each isoform is shown [41]. The melanopsin gene can generate, by alternate splicing, a long or a short isoform of the protein. Differences in the number of amino acids at the carboxyl terminus are what determine one form or another. The Long isoform consists of 521 aa and of 466 aa the Short one. M1 and M3 melanopsin ganglion cell subtypes co-express both isoforms, while M2 cells exclusively express the Long one [41].

It is also possible to perform a classification depending on the transcription factors expressed in ganglion cells. One of the members of the Brn3 family, Brn3b, allows us to appreciate if different subtypes of melanopsin cells are Brn3b positive or not. Brn3b transcription factor is necessary for the appropriate development of ganglion cells and suitable projection of their axons [42]. Its absence affects significantly the function of ganglion cells and, therefore, of melanopsin cells. Perhaps, the most important consequence is the loss of the pupillary light reflex, although the circadian activity regulation remains [43]. It has been reported that Brn3b is expressed on a small part of the M1 population, while Brn3a and Brn3c factors are not present in melanopsin ganglion cells.

The distribution of melanopsin cells in retina is very homogeneous and their dendritic trees (M1, M2, M3) cover the retina fully. However, in rat, populations of melanopsin ganglion cells have a higher density of cell bodies in the periphery, especially in the superior temporal quadrant [44, 45]. In other species, such as macaque, there is a similar distribution of cell bodies. It has also been found that dendritic arbors of these cells spread throughout the whole retina, except the fovea [36]. Previous morphological studies showed a more uniform distribution of the cell bodies in the retina [25]. This may be due to the labeling technique (X-gal) used in those studies, which does not reveal all subtypes of melanopsin ganglion cells present in the retina.

In spite of these efforts, subtypes of ipRGCs have not been completely defined yet, either by using high specificity and sensitivity melanopsin antibodies, or by genetic modification studies.

New techniques have helped to identify new morphological types of melanopsin ganglion cells. Thanks to the Cre/loxP system, which inserts reporter genes in melanopsin cells, two new subtypes have been detected: M4 and M5. These two subtypes could not be detected by conventional pathohistological methods, because they were not immunoreactive to antibodies against melanopsin [46]. However, with this technique, we are able to visualize the integrated marker in melanopsin cells [47]. Both cellular subtypes extend their dendrites along the inner sublamina (ON) of the IPL. The M4 ganglion cell has the largest soma of all melanopsin ganglion cells known. Its dendritic field is as vast and complex as that of M2 cells. However, its electrophysiological responses are small. M5 subtype cells have similar electrophysiological characteristics, although their soma size is one of the smallest [46]. Probably, the low photosensitive response is due to a minimal opsin presence. This could also explain why these subtypes cannot be detected by immunohistochemistry.

Up to date, ipRGCs are composed, at least, of five different subtypes. All these cells show projections to higher centers, sometimes well defined (M1 and M2; [25, 30]), and others still unknown (M3). See Figure 2 for a complete description.

Cellular Targets of ipRGCs

The origin of these studies was trying to explain why blind mice retained non-visual functions (as circadian photoentrainment). An important clue was given when mammals endogenous watch (the SCN) was understood [48]. Projections of ganglion cells to the SCN were studied by retrograde labeling. It was observed that "most RGCs that project to the SCN express melanopsin, and a majority of melanopsin-cointaining RGCs project to the SCN" [16]. Other interesting centers like the OPN (related to pupillary reflex control), IGL (related to circadian photoentrainment), and preoptic area (sleep control nucleus) were maintained in cone/rod less animals.

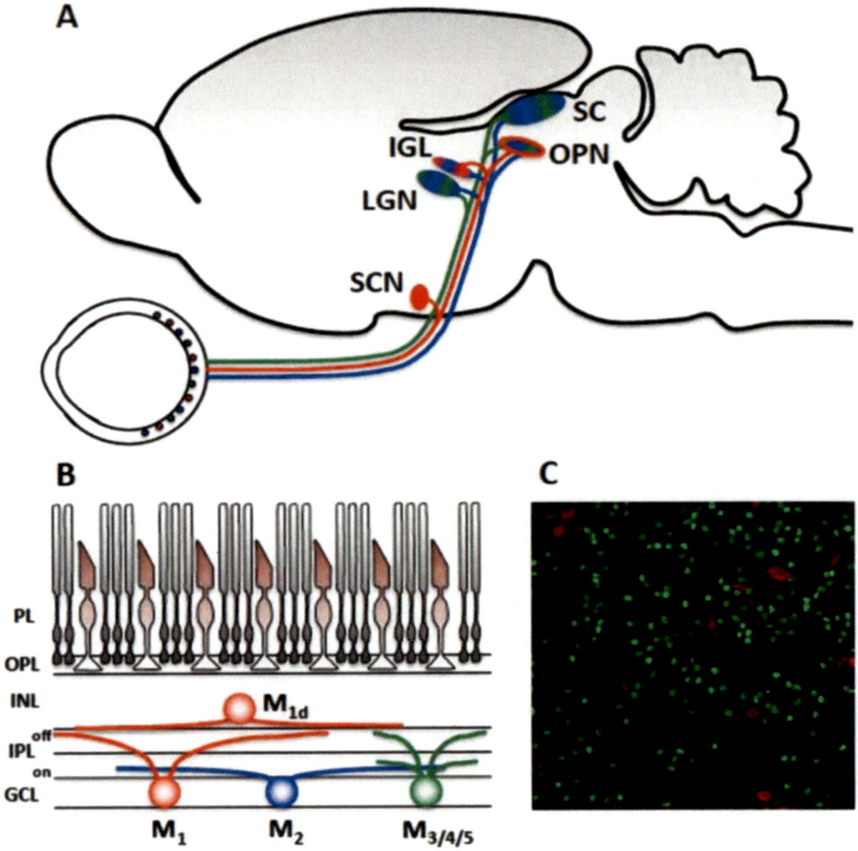

Figure 2. Morphological types of intrinsically photosensitive Retinal Ganglion Cells (ipRGC) and their main brain targets. **A**. Schematic representation of the mouse brain showing the nuclei innervated by ipRGC. SCN, suprachiasmatic nucleus; LGN: lateral geniculate nucleus; IGL: inter geniculate leaflet; OPN: olivary pretectal nucleus; SC: superior colliculus. **B**. Main ipRGC types in the mouse retina (M_1, M_{1d} [displaced], M_2, M_3, M_4, M_5) showing the characteristic dendritic arborization into the ON and OFF sublaminas of the inner plexiform layer (IPL). PL: photoreceptor layer; OPL: outer plexiform layer; INL: inner nuclear layer; GCL: ganglion cell layer. Color code of the M_1, M_{1d}, M_2, $M_{3/4/5}$ in B is used in A to show the main targets of each ipRGC subtype. **C**. Microphotograph of a small area of a flat mount retina showing ipRGC immunostained for melanopsin (red) in the GCL. Non-photosensitive Ganglion Cells are immunostained for Brn3a (green).

Some years later, other targets were identified, in total more than a dozen. Areas like ventral subparaventricular of hipotalamus, are involved in the disruption of motor activity when nightlife animals are exposed to light. Other important groups are the medial amygdala, the marginal lateral habenular nucleus, superior colliculus, and periaqueductal gray. Another prominently, but with fewer projections, is the dLGN (dorsal lateral geniculate nucleus) [25].

Projections to these nuclei have been better identified because Cre-dependent lines are more sensitive. This explains a greater labeling in the OPN core than in shell [46]. Also, electrophysiological recordings in the dLGN and the visual cortex have shown a melanopsin-mediated response. This raises the possibility that, through ipRGCs, a rudimentary form of vision is maintained in the absence of other photosensitive cells [49].

According to these studies, different subtypes have specific higher centers preferences. Those ipRGCs that stratify in the ON sublamina project to the SCN and OPN shell; whereas those others stratifying in the OFF sublamina do so to the OPN and dLGN [25, 30, 43, 46]. M3 cells projection center remains unidentified due to their low number.

FUNCTIONAL CHARACTERISTICS

Photoexcitation properties of ganglion cells are due to the melanopsin protein. In 2002, the work of Berson and collaborators revealed the intrinsic excitability of those cells whose target was the SCN. They discovered a small population of neurons at the retinal GCL by injecting fluorescent microspheres in the SCN that was retrogradely transported to the somas [7].

Interestingly, the responses in these cells are very different from those observed in rods and cones. While classical photoreceptors respond to light stimulation hyperpolarizing its membrane, Berson found that light induced an increase in conductance and membrane depolarization in melanopsin cells. It was very striking to find opposite physiological responses between classical photoreceptors and melanopsin cells, especially if we consider they share the characteristic of photoexcitation. Moreover, ipRGC responses to light, or depolarizations, occur even in the absence of rods and cones. Indeed, electrophysiological response of these cells is independent of classical photoreceptors, as it has been reported with different techniques. For example, by studying healthy retinas after performing a pharmacological blockade of cellular communication [7, 32]; or by analyzing the recordings in animals with retinal degeneration [40, 50]; or by recording isolated cells from human liver (HEK293) transfected with melanopsin [51-53]. The location of the photosensitive capacity in a few ganglion cells of the retina is the reason why these cells are called “intrinsically photosensitive Retinal Ganglion Cells or ipRGC”.

Functional studies of these cells by electrophysiological analysis have confirmed the existence of different ipRGCs subtypes. M1 and M2 cells show different sensitivity to the responses evoked by light, input resistance, depolarizing response in darkness and latency spikes [37]. The M3 subtype, in spite of remaining as a distinct morphological population, has similar physiological properties to the M2 subtype [38].

Sensitivity of melanopsin cells to light stimulation shows an important difference with rods and cones. In ipRGCs, sensitivity is very low and responses very slow. Several seconds are required to observe the peak response after the stimulus and many more to return to baseline. Response speed can be up to 20 times slower than in rods and about 100 times slower than in cones [54]. These properties are derived from the low density of melanopsin. Thus, intensity of stimulation must be very high (a relatively bright stimulus) to trigger light-dependent depolarizations in ipRGCs [55]. Low density of melanopsin in the retina can be explained by the low number of cells bearing melanopsin and the low presence of protein per mm^2 [56]. Melanopsin appears entirely localized in the plasma membrane of ipRGCs [57]; therefore a photon has less choice of being captured by melanopsin than by other photosensitive cells photopigments. All this is reflected in the low sensitivity of these cells [58]. However, the efficiency of photon absorption is as high as that of rods, and therefore both are capable of producing a response to a single photon [59]. By contrast, photosensitive machinery of cones requires about 100 photons to act efficiently [60].

Spectrum of Absorption

Once it was demonstrated that melanopsin was the protein that absorbed light, it was necessary to study which its absorption spectrum and its maximum absorption were. Earlier, pupillary reflex studies in blind mice (rd / rd cl) showed that pupillary constriction was produced within a range of wavelengths between 420-625 nm [61]. Later, it was found that the greater efficiency of melanopsin was between 460 – 480 nm**.** Today, we consider the maximal response is at 480 nm, deduced from the examination of non-image-forming visual functions (pupillary light response and circadian activity), as well as from the analysis of the purified protein, [51, 62]. Therefore, that value has been established by consensus as the most suitable for the activation of the new pigment.

As all known opsins, melanopsin has a wavelength filter function, which determines isomerization of the chromophore placed within, in response to a certain wavelength. The photopigment absorbance, or filtration process, has been defined by its biochemical nature. Based on that, it is considered that the pigment shows bistability, since responses have been detected both, at long wavelengths (520-600 nm), as well as at short wavelengths (420-480 nm) [32, 63]. Further, the responses due to stimulation by light of 480 nm are higher if the protein has been previously subjected to illumination at long wavelengths [64]. In these conditions, photon absorption and isomerization of the chromophore generates an intermediate structure, a balanced proportion of the relaxed form (Melanopsin) and the excited form (Metamelanopsin) [58]. New researches reported an additional form, extramelanopsin, whose function could be a remnant of potentially active molecule [65]. This intermediate state allows maintaining the photoresponse for many hours.

Mechanism of Phototransduction

ipRGCs photosensivity requires a vitamin A-based chromophore [53]. This has been demonstrated in mice lacking RPE65 (Rpe65-/ -), a protein needed to regenerate the chromophore through the pigment epithelium [66]. However, the composition of this chromophore is not entirely clear. The process opsins suffer after photon absorptions is retinoid chromophore isomerization. In conventional photoreceptors, the retinoid is 11-cis-retinal, which is photoisomerized to all-trans-retinal and activates a cascade through a G protein termed transducin (Gi/o).

The process continues with the activation of a phosphodiesterase (PDE) by transducin. The PDE acts reducing cGMP levels and, hence, promoting the closure of cGMP-dependent cation channels. This causes the hyperpolarizing response to a light stimulus observed in rods and cones. The new *retinal* (all trans) dissociates from the opsin and, thus, can be recycled into an active form (11 *cis*) by a series of reactions in the pigment epithelium.

Looking for the appropriate melanopsin isomer, several groups have used various potential molecules, 9 *cis*, 11 *cis*, 13 *cis* and all trans retinaldehyde. Although, all of them have demonstrated to be effective [55, 67], there are strong evidences that point out 11 *cis* retinal as the best chromophore for these cells [68].

The versatility showed in the use of retinal is another point in favor of melanopsin bistability. This opsin belongs to the superfamily of G protein-coupled receptors. This family keeps the chromophore conjugated to an amino acid of one of the transmembrane domains (a lysine of the domain VII) by a Schiff base [69].

Differences in Opsin Activation

Since melanopsin belongs to the same family as rhodopsin and cone-opsins (or color opsins); one would expect a similar activation mode in response to light. However, although the mechanism is not fully known, significant differences in the activation pathways of these chromophores have been identified.

The first difference arises from melanopsin interactions with a distinct type of G protein. In this case transducin is not involved, but another family member, Gq/G11 [70].

The next difference is in the type of enzyme coupled to the G protein; it is a phospholipase C (PLC), instead of a PDE. This fact generates a battery of potential second messengers whose final result will be the induction of the depolarizing currents. These second messengers may be diffusible, such as IP_3 (inositol triphosphate) and Ca^{2+}, or be attached to membranes, such as diacylglycerol and polyunsaturated fatty acids [71]. Although it is unclear which one is the main, it seems that, at least in *anurans* and *cephalochordata*, calcium is an important agent in phototransduction [60]. Effector channels suggested such depolarizations are transient receptor potential (TRP), whose opening allows the entry of cations to the cell cytoplasm.

The last major difference is the renovation of chromophore. Considering the distance between ganglion cells and pigment epithelial is quite large, the question to be asked is how the regeneration of the chromophore occurs. An explanation is given by the bistable nature of the protein. Because of this ability, melanopsin can change from one isomer to another (cis-trans) keeping its photoexcitable competitiveness. For this reason, melanopsin activity remains even when the pigment epithelium has no regenerative capacity [72, 73]. However, other studies have shown that in permanent darkness only 11-cis-retinal was isolated from the cell, and not a balance between the chromophores 11-cis and all-trans, as we would expect. In this case, it seems that a double regeneration, light-dependent and light-independent, of the chromophore is possible [68].

Relationships with Invertebrate

Peculiar features of melanopsin such as bistable nature, sensitivity peak at 480 nm, visual pigment coupled to Gq, PLC as Gq protein effector, IP_3 as second messenger, presence of TRP channels, and the depolarizing response to light, suggest a more close relationship with invertebrate than with vertebrate opsins. In fact, structural analysis of the protein reveals that the amino acid sequence has greater homology with invertebrates' opsins than with vertebrates' [74, 75]. The first ones are termed rhabdomeric opsins whereas the second ones are named ciliary opsins. Both lineages are originated from a common ancestor [76].

Melanopsin has been described primarily in cells belonging to the innermost layer of the retina. Both, in *Xenopus*, the species where it was discovered, and in a variety of mammals used in research, these cells have been described as ganglion cells. However, the presence of melanopsin in other mammalian retinal cell types has been documented, such as in human cones [77]. Far from mammals, in teleosts and birds, this opsin has been found in virtually all strata and all cell types of the retina [78, 79]. This variety of opsin locations, together with the distinct times of melanopsin cells differentiation, allow reaching an early sensitivity to light. In fact, the main melanopsin cells, the ganglion cells, differentiate around five weeks before birth [76, 80]. Therefore, ganglion cells are the first to be fully formed to integrate melanopsin. Specifically in mice, these cells acquire their earliest expression (between the eleventh and tenth embryonic day) [4]. From birth (P0), melanopsin can carry out the phototransduction of light signals to regulate non-image-forming functions. Therefore, melanopsin cells are considered one of the first retinal neurons acquiring functionality [81, 82].

Ontogeny

In early stages of animal ontogeny, melanopsin represents almost all of the photosensitive cells across the retina. These cells display a high number in the neonate and, according to several authors, decrease as the animal becomes an adult [83]. However, in other works, the gradual growth of the retina was considered, and the result was that melanopsin cell counts were constant for every individual [35]. These values are similar to those of previous studies in rat and mouse. In conclusion, there is no loss of melanopsin cells during growth.

Molecular melanopsin levels are influenced by ambient lighting conditions. Thus, when quantifying melanopsin expression in a light-dark cycle, this is higher in the hours of darkness than in the daylight hours [84, 85]. In rat, when the animal has been exposed to a long dark period, expression levels of melanopsin are high. If there has been a prolonged adaptation to constant light, messenger RNA levels and melanopsin immunoreactivity decrease markedly instead [86]. Also, some differences have been detected between M1 and M2 melanopsin cell subtypes. A change in opsin levels was observed in condition of darkness for the M1 subtype, whereas the M2 subtype maintains opsin levels constant [87]. This fact establishes a direct relationship between classical photoreceptors and ipRGCs. In this regard, it has been shown that there is a dependence of melanopsin expression on rod and cone inputs, at least in the M1 subtype. This dependence is such that the loss of rods and cones results in the loss of melanopsin circadian expression [88]. However, modifications in its expression to a homogeneous long-term lighting are kept. Also, increased mRNA expression and melanopsin immunoreactivity in newborns (P5), where classical photoreceptors are not yet functionally developed, have been demonstrated [86].

Intraretinal Connections of ipRGCs

Extrinsic signaling to ipRGCs denotes a communication with other retinal cell types. Since rods and cones may influence the activation of melanopsin cells, a direct signaling pathway between them must exist. Several studies have shown that ipRGCs communicate with INL cells through their processes in both sublayers of the IPL. Electron microscopy techniques have allowed the description of the retinal circuit that connects ON bipolar cells with ipRGCs [57]. Other techniques that use genetically modified animal models (carrying fluorescent reporters under the control of specific promoters) have facilitated the discovery of connections with amacrine and bipolar cells [31, 34, 89]. The use of confocal microscopy and subsequent analysis of the 3D images restored by sophisticated software have also provided information on the connections between melanopsin cells and ON bipolar cells and dopaminergic amacrine cells [90]. The main pathway of these inputs from photoreceptors is the pathway of rods through type II amacrine cells (AII). These amacrine cells are necessary to carry the signal from rod bipolar cells to ganglion cells before leaving the eyeball. However, the connection points of AII cells with ipRGCs vary for each cell subtype. Before analyzing the possible contacts, we have to remember that the M2, M4 and M5 subtypes extend their dendrites throughout the sublamina ON of IPL. In contrast, the M1 subtype spreads its dendritic tree in the sublamina OFF (so one would expect connections to OFF bipolar cells). Despite this, M1 subtype receives inputs from ON cone bipolar cells through the sublamina OFF [89]. Indeed, there is evidence of ribbon synapses between ON bipolar cells and ipRGCs in the sublamina OFF.

In the longest circuit, the signal goes sequentially from a rod bipolar cell to AII amacrine cell, to cone bipolar cell and, finally, to M1 type cells. There is a second pathway that leads signals from rods to ipRGCs through ON cone bipolar cells. The third pathway employs the existing communication between classic photoreceptors. Through this synapse the signal goes from rod to cone and hence to cone bipolar cell (type ON) to finally contact the ipRGC [91]. The last circuit, if somewhat unusual, connects rods with the M1 subtype through the rod bipolar cells [90].

Melanopsin and Non-Image-Forming Visual Functions

Melanopsin plays a fundamental role in non-image-forming visual functions (see Figure 3). Its importance lays in the modulatory role of animal behavior. Among the visual tasks in which ipRGCs have a major role are:

- The pupillary light reflex function is adjusting the size of the pupil to optimize the amount of light reaching rods and cones. This reflex is triggered by the light acting on any of the photoreceptors of the retina [92]. However, ipRGCs are enough to maintain the pupillary reflex. The most effective response is observed at 479 nm [61].
- The regulation of circadian rhythms. Living beings have their daily actions, and even many of their metabolic processes, conditioned to a particular time of the day. Our body maintains the rhythms of various functions through an endogenous clock. This is set by signals (*zeitgeber*, discussed earlier in this document) from the external environment, such as light. Without an external signal indicative of the time of day (light / dark), our endogenous clock is able to keep a

daily rhythm for different bodily functions. One of these functions is motor activity that in nocturnal animals (such as mice, used in laboratory) takes place in the hours of darkness. This activity is observed even in certain blindness types. In these situations there is a lack of classical photoreceptors but, as melanopsin is still present, ipRGCs become the primary responsible to command or regulate certain behaviors [93].

It is possible to evaluate the ability to regulate circadian activity in two ways. The first one is by applying a pulse of light at the maximal activity hours of the animal. When the animal perceives light, stops its activity (in nocturnal animals) and continues when the flash of light is finished. This is called photoentrainment. If this pulse of light causes advancement in activity in the following days this is a *positive phase-shift*. On the contrary, if the activity is delayed we are talking about a *negative phase-shift* [94]. The second way is to modify the characteristics of the light to change animal behavior. This is called masking, since light can hide or mask the signal coming from the endogenous clock [95].

- Sleep regulation. In mouse (nocturnal animal), surprisingly, a pulse of light amid the dark phase causes sleepiness [96]; while a moment of darkness during the light phase induces awakening. This induction of sleep seems to be associated with the expression of c-fos [97, 98]. It has also been observed that these modulations are lost in melanopsin *knock out* mouse.
- Suppression of pineal melatonin. Melatonin is a hormone that is elevated in blood in the hours of darkness and suppressed during the day by light stimulus. One of the targets of ipRGCs is related to the production of melatonin. Thus, melanopsin is closely related to the levels of melatonin.

There are animals whose only photosensitive cells are ipRGCs. As we would expect, in these animals the non-image-forming visual functions are maintained. However, lack of melanopsin does not completely eliminate these functions, but reduces them. The cancellation of these functions occurs only when the ganglion cells that project to their control centers are lost. Elimination of these cells can be experimentally achieved by genetic engineering techniques such as the conditional expression of certain toxin receptors in melanopsin cells [47, 99]. Axons that leave the eyeball and are not involved in image formation form the nerve cord known as retinohypothalamic tract (RHT).

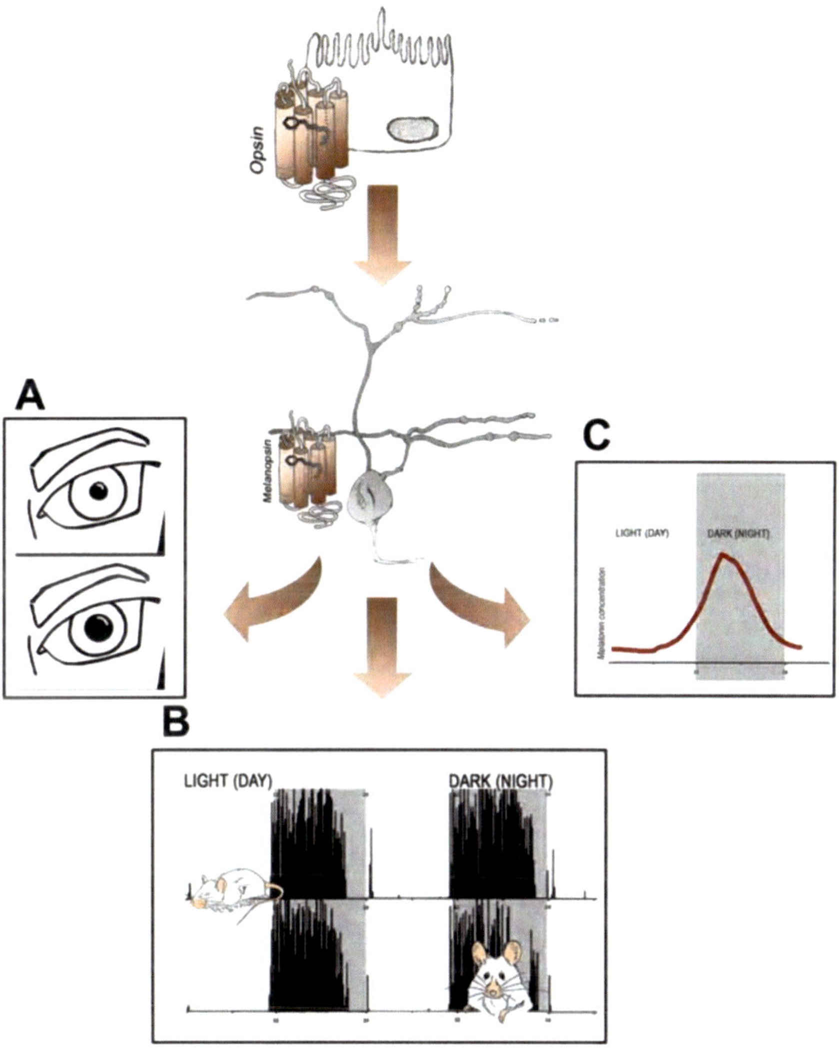

Figure 3. Intrinsically photosensitive Retinal Ganglion Cells. These cells are an evolved form of rhabdomeric cells. Their functions are due to the expression of melanopsin, and are responsible for the pupillary reflex or iris constriction (**A**); regulation of circadian rhythms (nocturnal animals such as mice show activity during the night and rest during daytime) (**B**); and suppression of pineal melatonin during daytime (**C**).

Many of the melanopsin cell targets display a peptide called pituitary adenylyl cyclase-activating protein (PACAP) [100], which had previously been documented in the CNS [101]. The peptide is also present in the ganglion cell somas found both, in the GCL as well as in the INL, and also in the ganglion cell processes extended through the IPL [102]. Likewise, the presence of PACAP has been confirmed in the human RHT [103].

PHYLOGENY OF IPRGCS

The melanopsin cell plays a functional role in our retinas alongside "traditional photoreceptors", rods and cones. This cell is amazing, not only for its functional role in behavioral processes, but also by its very nature. Its characteristics and features place these cells away from other light-sensitive cells in vertebrates, and approach them to invertebrates instead. Indeed, there are important differences between perception organs in different *subphyllum*: *vertebrata* and *invertebrata.*

Therefore, we can ask ourselves: why a cell belonging to such a different organism is found in our eye? How different are the sensory organs of all of them?

Several theories try to explain how the variety of visual organs has been developed along evolution. This variety could occur independently during evolution or, conversely, from a common origin. The first theory is based on the different developmental processes that ensue in the eye of invertebrates and vertebrates. Moreover, both retinas come from different embrionary layers, the neuroectoderm (vertebrates) and the ectoderm (invertebrates). Even genetic factors are different in the *invertebrata* and *vertebrata* eye ontogeny [104].

The second theory, by contrast, points to the existence of a precursor for all current models. One of its arguments is based on the presence of certain genes in eye development, both in vertebrate and invertebrate [105]. Therefore, these genes may have belonged to a previous organism and, after branch division, remain in different species (orthologous genes). Thus, both eyes would be generated by a repertoire of orthologous genes in similar areas of the embryo [104].

Regarding sensorial organs, an important difference between vertebrates and invertebrates is the type of photosensitive cell. There are two types described: rhabdomeric and ciliary photoreceptors. The former are exclusively related to arthropods. In other evolutionary lines like *Protostomes (*mollusks and annelids), rhabdomeric are the predominant ones. Their mechanism of action is associated with a Gq protein, which initiates the phototransduction cascade. Ciliary and rhabdomeric photoreceptors are present in *Deuterostomes*. Nevertheless, vertebrate organisms had been related only to ciliary cells [76]. This drastic separation between models ended when melanopsin was found in the eyes of mammals and other vertebrates. Moreover, the *phylum Cephalochordata* also showed the presence of both types of cells, particularly in *Branchiostoma*, an organism previous to the onset of the *vertebrata subphylum* [63]. The separation point of the two cell types remains unkonwn. In this line, the work of Ardent and collaborators identified the *Urbilateria* species as the common ancestor of both cell types. This species belongs to *superphylum Bilateria*, which is the origin of all actual species with bilateral symmetry [106] (See Figure 4).

From *Urbilateria*, organisms have been exposed to different environmental conditions that have modified their photosensitive structures. Even more, the photosensitive molecules of the different cells (ciliary or rhabdomeric) have evolved through small protein modifications. Thus, we find photosensitive proteins (opsin) with different wavelength ranges of excitation. In this regard, melanopsin cells (rhabdomeric nature) show an excitation spectrum around the blue light. Adaptation to this type of light is very useful for species in whose habitat blue light is the predominant, for example aquatic species [107].

With the emergence of vertebrate species new opsins appeared. In vertebrates, these proteins were added to the pre-existing opsins of invertebrates. However, the melanopsin gene (Opn4) is not uniform in all vertebrate species. There are two melanopsin genes in vertebrates: mammalian-like melanopsin (Opn4m) and xenopus-like melanopsin (Opn4x). Mammals express Opn4m only in the retina, specifically in a neuronal type (retinal ganglion cells). However, non-mammals may express one or both genes in different tissues: retina (various cell types), brain, and pineal gland. Five different melanopsins exist in the *subclass Teleostei* : Opn4x1, Opn4x2, Opn4m1, Opn4m2 and Opn4m3. In teleost species, the vast majority of retinal cell types express some type of melanopsin [108].

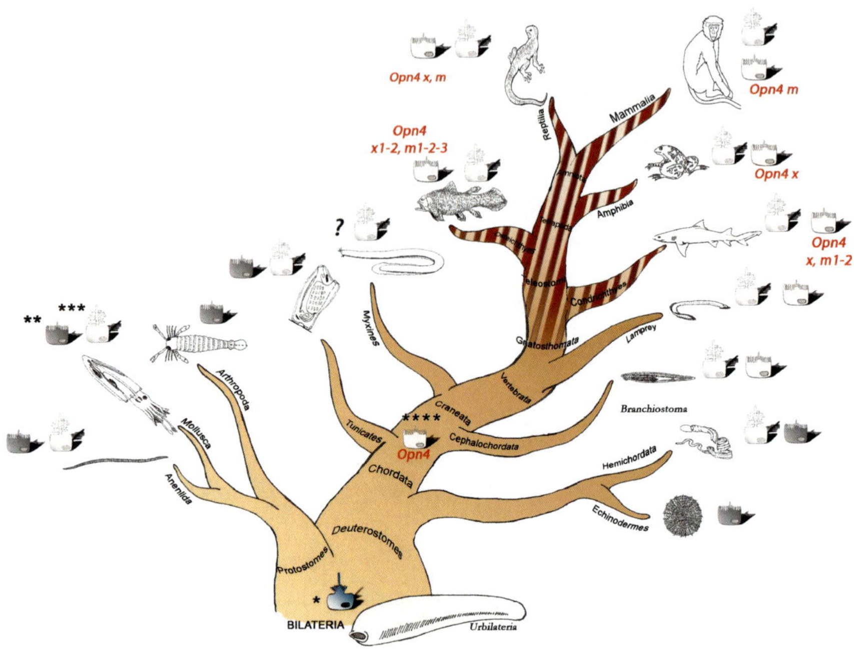

Figure 4. Phylogenetic tree of photoexcitable cells. The origin of all the *Bilateria* species was *Urbilateria* (*). Later, bilateral symmetry organisms emerged. In such organisms two types of light-sensitive cells have been identified. Indeed, *Urbilateria* could possess either the two cellular types or a precursor thereof. These two types of light-sensitive cells are the rhabdomeric cells (**) and the ciliary cells (***). *Superphyllum protostomata* shows both types, although the rhabdomeric type is more relevant. Also *Superphyllum deuterostomata, phylum chordate* presents groups with both cell types, por ejemplo *urochordata (tunicata), cephalocordata (amphioxus branquiostoma belcheri*) y vertebrata. The brush cell (****) indicates the evolutionary point where it seems that melanopsin (photoexcitable protein) could arise. There are several types of melanopsin that may appear in one or several species. So while amphibians only have Opn4x, mammals only have the form Opn4m. However, other species evolutionarily older have many isoforms of such protein. For example, in the *Osteichthyes* superclass (specifically the *Sarcopterygii* class, *teleostei* subclass) up to 5 different types of opsins (Opn4 x1, x2, m1, m2, m3) have been reported. It seems that the divergence of the gene Opn4 in their forms x and m occurred 320 million years ago (dashed lines of the phylogenetic tree).

NEW HORIZONS IN RESEARCH

Nature never ceases to amaze. The discovery of new photosensitive cells involved in behavioral and non-image-forming visual functions has opened new pathways of research. Particularly interesting is the fact that the cell involved in these functions maintains a bridge with invertebrates. Some questions remain unanswered, for instance, why keeping that photoexcitable cell if more evolved ones exist?

The new pathways of research try to provide solutions to everyday problems. For example, seasonal disorders related to the level of light [109]. Also, the types of lighting in night work can be improved if the role and functioning of melanopsin cells are known, thus improving life quality of these workers. Currently, even age related retinal disorders seem to be associated to the type of light and the functional role of ipRGCs [110]. A very wide variety of diseases are being analyzed from the perspective of the functional role of ipRGCs, like for example migraines and certain types of neoplasia [111].

REFERENCES

[1] Darwin, C. (1859). On the origin of species by means of natural selection, or The preservation of favoured races in the struggle for life. London, *J. Murray. ix, 1*, 502 p.

[2] Sharma, V. K. & Chandrashekaran, M. K. (2005). Zeitgebers (time cues) for biological clocks. *Current Science*, *89*(7), 1136-1146.

[3] Pandey, S., et al. (1994). Cytoplasmic retinal localization of an evolutionary homolog of the visual pigments. *Exp Eye Res*, *58*(5), 605-13.

[4] Tarttelin, E. E., et al. (2003). Neuropsin (Opn5): a novel opsin identified in mammalian neural tissue. *FEBS Lett*, *554*(3), 410-6.

[5] Sun, H., et al. (1997). Peropsin, a novel visual pigment-like protein located in the apical microvilli of the retinal pigment epithelium. *Proc Natl Acad Sci U S A*, *94*(18), 9893-8.

[6] Provencio, I., et al. (1998). Melanopsin: An opsin in melanophores, brain, and eye. *Proc Natl Acad Sci U S A*, *95*(1), 340-5.

[7] Berson, D. M., Dunn, F. A. & Takao, M. (2002). Phototransduction by retinal ganglion cells that set the circadian clock. *Science*, *295*(5557), 1070-3.

[8] Keeler, C. E. (1927). Iris movements in blind mice. *American Journal of Physiology*. *81*(1), 107-112.
[9] Morgan, W. W. & Kamp, C. W. (1980). Dopaminergic amacrine neurons of rat retinas with photoreceptor degeneration continue to respond to light. *Life Sci*, *26*(19), 1619-26.
[10] Czeisler, C. A., et al. (1995). Suppression of melatonin secretion in some blind patients by exposure to bright light. *N Engl J Med*, *332*(1), 6-11.
[11] Lucas, R. J., et al. (1999). Regulation of the mammalian pineal by non-rod, non-cone, ocular photoreceptors. *Science*, *284*(5413), 505-7.
[12] Ebihara, S. & Tsuji, K. (1980). Entrainment of the circadian activity rhythm to the light cycle: effective light intensity for a Zeitgeber in the retinal degenerate C3H mouse and the normal C57BL mouse. *Physiol Behav*, *24*(3), 523-7.
[13] Foster, R. G., et al. (1991). Circadian photoreception in the retinally degenerate mouse (rd/rd). *J Comp Physiol A*, *169*(1), 39-50.
[14] Provencio, I., et al. (1994). Visual and circadian responses to light in aged retinally degenerate mice. *Vision Res*, *34*(14), 1799-806.
[15] Provencio, I., et al. (2000). A novel human opsin in the inner retina. *J Neurosci*, *20*(2), 600-5.
[16] Gooley, J. J., et al. (2001). Melanopsin in cells of origin of the retinohypothalamic tract. *Nat Neurosci*, *4*(12), p. 1165.
[17] Hattar, S., et al. (2002). Melanopsin-containing retinal ganglion cells: architecture, projections, and intrinsic photosensitivity. *Science*, *295*(5557), 1065-70.
[18] Thresher, R. J., et al. (1998). Role of mouse cryptochrome blue-light photoreceptor in circadian photoresponses. *Science*, *282*(5393), 1490-4.
[19] Panda, S., et al. (2003). Melanopsin is required for non-image-forming photic responses in blind mice. *Science*, *301*(5632), 525-7.
[20] Hattar, S., et al. (2003). Melanopsin and rod-cone photoreceptive systems account for all major accessory visual functions in mice. *Nature*, *424*(6944), 76-81.
[21] Van Gelder, R. N., et al. (2003). Reduced pupillary light responses in mice lacking cryptochromes. Science, 299(5604), p. 222.
[22] Filipek, S., et al. (2003). G protein-coupled receptor rhodopsin: a prospectus. *Annu Rev Physiol.*, *65*, 851-79.
[23] Schadel, S. A., et al. (2003). Ligand channeling within a G-protein-coupled receptor. The entry and exit of retinals in native opsin. *J Biol Chem*, *278*(27), 24896-903.

[24] Drager, U. C. & J. F. Olsen. (1980). Origins of crossed and uncrossed retinal projections in pigmented and albino mice. *J Comp Neurol*, *191*(3), 383-412.

[25] Hattar, S., et al. (2006). Central projections of melanopsin-expressing retinal ganglion cells in the mouse. *J Comp Neurol*, *497*(3), 326-49.

[26] Gonzalez-Menendez, I., et al. (2010). Postnatal development and functional adaptations of the melanopsin photoreceptive system in the albino mouse retina. *Invest Ophthalmol Vis Sci*, *51*(9), 4840-7.

[27] Berson, D. M., Castrucci, A. M. & Provencio, I. (2010). Morphology and mosaics of melanopsin-expressing retinal ganglion cell types in mice. *J Comp Neurol*, *518*(13), 2405-22.

[28] Provencio, I., Rollag, M. D. & Castrucci, A. M. (2002). Photoreceptive net in the mammalian retina. This mesh of cells may explain how some blind mice can still tell day from night. *Nature*, *415*(6871), p. 493.

[29] Sand, A., Schmidt, T. M. & Kofuji, P. (2012). Diverse types of ganglion cell photoreceptors in the mammalian retina. *Prog Retin Eye Res*, *31*(4), 287-302.

[30] Baver, S. B., Pickard, G. E. & Sollars, P. J. (2008). Two types of melanopsin retinal ganglion cell differentially innervate the hypothalamic suprachiasmatic nucleus and the olivary pretectal nucleus. *Eur J Neurosci*, *27*(7), 1763-70.

[31] Viney, T. J., et al. (2007). Local retinal circuits of melanopsin-containing ganglion cells identified by transsynaptic viral tracing. *Curr Biol*, *17*(11), 981-8.

[32] Schmidt, T. M., Taniguchi, K. & Kofuji, P. (2008). Intrinsic and extrinsic light responses in melanopsin-expressing ganglion cells during mouse development. *J Neurophysiol*, *100*(1), 371-84.

[33] Schmidt, T. M., Chen, S. K. & Hattar, S. (2011). Intrinsically photosensitive retinal ganglion cells: many subtypes, diverse functions. *Trends Neurosci*, *34*(11), 572-80.

[34] Muller, L. P., et al. (2010). Tracer coupling of intrinsically photosensitive retinal ganglion cells to amacrine cells in the mouse retina. *J Comp Neurol*, *518*(23), 4813-24.

[35] Gonzalez-Menendez, I., et al. (2010). No loss of melanopsin-expressing ganglion cells detected during postnatal development of the mouse retina. *Histol Histopathol*, *25*(1), 73-82.

[36] Dacey, D. M., et al. (2005). Melanopsin-expressing ganglion cells in primate retina signal colour and irradiance and project to the LGN. *Nature*, *433*(7027), 749-54.

[37] Schmidt, T. M. & Kofuji, P. (2009). Functional and morphological differences among intrinsically photosensitive retinal ganglion cells. *J Neurosci*, *29*(2), 476-82.

[38] Schmidt, T. M. & Kofuji, P. (2011). Structure and function of bistratified intrinsically photosensitive retinal ganglion cells in the mouse. *J Comp Neurol*, *519*(8), 1492-504.

[39] Sekaran, S., et al. (2003). Calcium imaging reveals a network of intrinsically light-sensitive inner-retinal neurons. *Curr Biol*, *13*(15), 1290-8.

[40] Tu, D. C., et al. (2005). Physiologic diversity and development of intrinsically photosensitive retinal ganglion cells. *Neuron*, *48*(6), 987-99.

[41] Pires, S. S., et al. (2009). Differential expression of two distinct functional isoforms of melanopsin (Opn4) in the mammalian retina. *J Neurosci*, *29*(39), 12332-42.

[42] Badea, T. C., et al. (2009). Distinct roles of transcription factors brn3a and brn3b in controlling the development, morphology, and function of retinal ganglion cells. *Neuron*, *61*(6), 852-64.

[43] Chen, S. K., Badea, T. C. & Hattar, S. (2011). Photoentrainment and pupillary light reflex are mediated by distinct populations of ipRGCs. *Nature*, *476*(7358), 92-5.

[44] Galindo-Romero, C., et al. (2013). Number and spatial distribution of intrinsically photosensitive retinal ganglion cells in the adult albino rat. *Exp Eye Res*, *108*, 84-93.

[45] Hughes, S., et al. (2013). Nonuniform distribution and spectral tuning of photosensitive retinal ganglion cells of the mouse retina. *Curr Biol*, *23*(17), 1696-701.

[46] Ecker, J. L., et al. (2010). Melanopsin-expressing retinal ganglion-cell photoreceptors: cellular diversity and role in pattern vision. *Neuron*, *67*(1), 49-60.

[47] Hatori, M., et al. (2008). Inducible ablation of melanopsin-expressing retinal ganglion cells reveals their central role in non-image forming visual responses. *PLoS One*, *3*(6), p. e2451.

[48] Moore, R. Y. (2007). Suprachiasmatic nucleus in sleep-wake regulation. *Sleep Med*, *8* Suppl 3, 27-33.

[49] Brown, T. M., et al. (2010). Melanopsin contributions to irradiance coding in the thalamo-cortical visual system. *PLoS Biol*, *8*(12), p. e1000558.

[50] Lin, B., et al. (2008). Restoration of visual function in retinal degeneration mice by ectopic expression of melanopsin. *Proc Natl Acad Sci U S A*, *105*(41), 16009-14.
[51] Qiu, X., et al. (2005). Induction of photosensitivity by heterologous expression of melanopsin. *Nature*, *433*(7027), 745-9.
[52] Kumbalasiri, T., et al. (2007). Melanopsin triggers the release of internal calcium stores in response to light. *Photochem Photobiol*, *83*(2), 273-9.
[53] Giesbers, M. E., et al. (2008). Functional expression, targeting and Ca2+ signaling of a mouse melanopsin-eYFP fusion protein in a retinal pigment epithelium cell line. *Photochem Photobiol*, *84*(4), p. 990-5.
[54] Mata, N. L., et al. (2002). Isomerization and oxidation of vitamin a in cone-dominant retinas: a novel pathway for visual-pigment regeneration in daylight. *Neuron*, *36*(1), 69-80.
[55] Panda, S., et al. (2005). Illumination of the melanopsin signaling pathway. *Science*, *307*(5709), 600-4.
[56] Brown, T. M. & Lucas, R. J. (2009). Melanopsin phototransduction: great excitement over a poor catch. *Curr Biol*, *19*(6), p. R256-7.
[57] Belenky, M. A., et al. (2003). Melanopsin retinal ganglion cells receive bipolar and amacrine cell synapses. *J Comp Neurol*, *460*(3), 380-93.
[58] Berson, D. M. (2007). Phototransduction in ganglion-cell photoreceptors. *Pflugers Arch*, *454*(5), 849-55.
[59] Do, M. T., et al. (2009). Photon capture and signalling by melanopsin retinal ganglion cells. *Nature*, *457*(7227), 281-7.
[60] Do, M. T. & Yau, K. W. (2010). Intrinsically photosensitive retinal ganglion cells. *Physiol Rev*, *90*(4), 1547-81.
[61] Lucas, R. J., Douglas, R. H. & Foster, R. G. (2001). Characterization of an ocular photopigment capable of driving pupillary constriction in mice. *Nat Neurosci*, *4*(6), 621-6.
[62] Newman, L. A., et al. (2003). Melanopsin forms a functional short-wavelength photopigment. *Biochemistry*, *42*(44), 12734-8.
[63] Koyanagi, M., et al. (2005). Cephalochordate melanopsin: evolutionary linkage between invertebrate visual cells and vertebrate photosensitive retinal ganglion cells. *Curr Biol*, *15*(11), 1065-9.
[64] Mure, L. S., et al. (2007). Melanopsin-dependent nonvisual responses: evidence for photopigment bistability in vivo. *J Biol Rhythms*, *22*(5), 411-24.
[65] Matsuyama, T., et al. (2012). Photochemical properties of mammalian melanopsin. *Biochemistry*, *51*(27), 5454-62.

[66] Fu, Y., et al. (2005). Intrinsically photosensitive retinal ganglion cells detect light with a vitamin A-based photopigment, melanopsin. *Proc Natl Acad Sci U S A*, *102*(29), 10339-44.

[67] Melyan, Z., et al. (2005). Addition of human melanopsin renders mammalian cells photoresponsive. *Nature*, *433*(7027), 741-5.

[68] Walker, M. T., et al. (2008). Photochemistry of retinal chromophore in mouse melanopsin. *Proc Natl Acad Sci U S A*, *105*(26), 8861-5.

[69] Davies, W. L., Foster, R. G., & Hankins, M. W. (2012). Focus on molecules: melanopsin. *Exp Eye Res*, *97*(1), 161-2.

[70] Terakita, A., et al. (2008). Expression and comparative characterization of Gq-coupled invertebrate visual pigments and melanopsin. *J Neurochem*, *105*(3), 883-90.

[71] Graham, D. M., et al. (2008). Melanopsin ganglion cells use a membrane-associated rhabdomeric phototransduction cascade. *J Neurophysiol*, *99*(5), 2522-32.

[72] Tu, D. C., et al. (2006). Inner retinal photoreception independent of the visual retinoid cycle. *Proc Natl Acad Sci U S A*, *103*(27), 10426-31.

[73] Doyle, S. E., et al. (2006). Nonvisual light responses in the Rpe65 knockout mouse: rod loss restores sensitivity to the melanopsin system. *Proc Natl Acad Sci U S A*, *103*(27), 10432-7.

[74] Bellingham, J. & Foster, R. G. (2002). Opsins and mammalian photoentrainment. *Cell Tissue Res*,. *309*(1), 57-71.

[75] Hankins, M. W., Peirson, S. N. & Foster, R. G. (2008). Melanopsin: an exciting photopigment. *Trends Neurosci*, *31*(1), 27-36.

[76] Lamb, T. D., Collin, S. P. & Pugh, Jr. E. N. (2007). Evolution of the vertebrate eye: opsins, photoreceptors, retina and eye cup. *Nat Rev Neurosci*, *8*(12), 960-76.

[77] Dkhissi-Benyahya, O., et al. (2006). Immunohistochemical evidence of a melanopsin cone in human retina. *Invest Ophthalmol Vis Sci*, *47*(4), 1636-41.

[78] Cheng, N. Tsunenari, T. & Yau, K. W. (2009). Intrinsic light response of retinal horizontal cells of teleosts. *Nature*, *460*(7257), 899-903.

[79] Chaurasia, S. S., et al. (2005). Molecular cloning, localization and circadian expression of chicken melanopsin (Opn4): differential regulation of expression in pineal and retinal cell types. *J Neurochem*, *92*(1), 158-70.

[80] Reese, B. E. (2011). Development of the retina and optic pathway. *Vision Res*, *51*(7), 613-32.

[81] Johnson, J., et al. (2010). Melanopsin-dependent light avoidance in neonatal mice. *Proc Natl Acad Sci U S A*, *107*(40), 17374-8.

[82] Renna, J. M., Weng, S. & Berson, D. M. (2011). Light acts through melanopsin to alter retinal waves and segregation of retinogeniculate afferents. *Nat Neurosci*, *14*(7), 827-9.

[83] Hannibal, J. & Fahrenkrug, J. (2004). Melanopsin containing retinal ganglion cells are light responsive from birth. *Neuroreport*, *15*(15), 2317-20.

[84] Sakamoto, K., et al. (2005). Dopamine regulates melanopsin mRNA expression in intrinsically photosensitive retinal ganglion cells. *Eur J Neurosci*, *22*(12), 3129-36.

[85] Mathes, A., et al. (2007). Daily profile in melanopsin transcripts depends on seasonal lighting conditions in the rat retina. *J Neuroendocrinol*, *19*(12), 952-7.

[86] Hannibal, J., Georg, B. & Fahrenkrug, J. (2007). Melanopsin changes in neonatal albino rat independent of rods and cones. *Neuroreport*, *18*(1), 81-5.

[87] Gonzalez-Menendez, I., et al. (2009). Daily rhythm of melanopsin-expressing cells in the mouse retina. *Front Cell Neurosci*, *3*, p. 3.

[88] Sakamoto, K., Liu, C. & Tosini, G. (2004). Classical photoreceptors regulate melanopsin mRNA levels in the rat retina. *J Neurosci*,. *24*(43), 9693-7.

[89] Dumitrescu, O. N., et al. (2009). Ectopic retinal ON bipolar cell synapses in the OFF inner plexiform layer: contacts with dopaminergic amacrine cells and melanopsin ganglion cells. *J Comp Neurol*, *517*(2), 226-44.

[90] Ostergaard, J., Hannibal, J. & Fahrenkrug, J. (2007). Synaptic contact between melanopsin-containing retinal ganglion cells and rod bipolar cells. *Invest Ophthalmol Vis Sci*, *48*(8), 3812-20.

[91] Weng, S., Estevez, M. E. & Berson, D. M. (2013). Mouse ganglion-cell photoreceptors are driven by the most sensitive rod pathway and by both types of cones. *PLoS One*, *8*(6), p. e66480.

[92] Park, J. C., et al. (2011). Toward a clinical protocol for assessing rod, cone, and melanopsin contributions to the human pupil response. *Invest Ophthalmol Vis Sci*, *52*(9), 6624-35.

[93] Ruby, N. F., et al. (2002). Role of melanopsin in circadian responses to light. *Science*, *298*(5601), 2211-3.

[94] Panda, S., et al. (2002). Melanopsin (Opn4) requirement for normal light-induced circadian phase shifting. *Science*, *298*(5601), 2213-6.

[95] Thompson, S., et al. (2008). Classical and melanopsin photoreception in irradiance detection: negative masking of locomotor activity by light. *Eur J Neurosci*, *27*(8), 1973-9.

[96] Lupi, D., et al. (2008). The acute light-induction of sleep is mediated by OPN4-based photoreception. *Nat Neurosci*, *11*(9), 1068-73.

[97] Lupi, D., et al. (2006). Light-evoked FOS induction within the suprachiasmatic nuclei (SCN) of melanopsin knockout (Opn4-/-) mice: a developmental study. *Chronobiol Int*, *23*(1-2), 167-79.

[98] Pickard, G. E., et al. (2009). Light-induced fos expression in intrinsically photosensitive retinal ganglion cells in melanopsin knockout (opn4) mice. *PLoS One*, *4*(3), p. e4984.

[99] Goz, D., et al. (2008). Targeted destruction of photosensitive retinal ganglion cells with a saporin conjugate alters the effects of light on mouse circadian rhythms. *PLoS One*, *3*(9), p. e3153.

[100] Hannibal, J., et al. (2001). Light-dependent induction of cFos during subjective day and night in PACAP-containing ganglion cells of the retinohypothalamic tract. *J Biol Rhythms*, *16*(5), 457-70.

[101] Hannibal, J., et al. (1995). Gene expression of pituitary adenylate cyclase activating polypeptide (PACAP) in the rat hypothalamus. *Regul Pept*,. *55*(2), 133-48.

[102] Hannibal, J., et al. (2002). The photopigment melanopsin is exclusively present in pituitary adenylate cyclase-activating polypeptide-containing retinal ganglion cells of the retinohypothalamic tract. *J Neurosci*, *22*(1), p. RC191.

[103] Hannibal, J., et al. (2004). Melanopsin is expressed in PACAP-containing retinal ganglion cells of the human retinohypothalamic tract. *Invest Ophthalmol Vis Sci*, *45*(11), 4202-9.

[104] Bailey, T. J., et al. (2004). Regulation of vertebrate eye development by Rx genes. *Int J Dev Biol*, *48*(8-9), 761-70.

[105] Gehring, W. J. (2004). Historical perspective on the development and evolution of eyes and photoreceptors. *Int J Dev Biol*, *48*(8-9), 707-17.

[106] Arendt, D. & Wittbrodt, J. (2001). Reconstructing the eyes of Urbilateria. *Philos Trans R Soc Lond B Biol Sci*,. *356*(1414), 1545-63.

[107] Davies, W. I., et al. (2012). Evolution and functional characterisation of melanopsins in a deep-sea chimaera (elephant shark, Callorhinchus milii). *PLoS One*, *7*(12), p. e51276.

[108] Borges, R., et al. (2012). The role of gene duplication and unconstrained selective pressures in the melanopsin gene family evolution and vertebrate circadian rhythm regulation. *PLoS One*, *7*(12), p. e52413.

[109] Roecklein, K. A., et al. (2009). A missense variant (P10L) of the melanopsin (OPN4) gene in seasonal affective disorder. *J Affect Disord, 114*(1-3), 279-85.

[110] Herbst, K., et al. (2012). Intrinsically photosensitive retinal ganglion cell function in relation to age: a pupillometric study in humans with special reference to the age-related optic properties of the lens. *BMC Ophthalmol*, *12*, p. 4.

[111] Davis, S., Mirick, D. K. & Stevens, R. G. (2001). Night shift work, light at night, and risk of breast cancer. *J Natl Cancer Inst*, *93*(20), 1557-62.

In: Ganglion Cells
Editor: Liora G. Vlastimil

ISBN: 978-1-63117-432-2

Chapter 3

DETAILED INSIGHTS INTO FUNCTIONAL RETINAL NEURODEGENERATION OF AGED DBA/2J GLAUCOMA MICE

Sven Schnichels[1] and Peter Heiduschka[2*]
[1]Centre for Ophthalmology, University Eye Hospital, Tübingen, Germany
[2]University of Münster Eye Hospital, Münster, Germany

ABSTRACT

The DBA/2J mouse is a common animal model of glaucoma. The intraocular pressure increases with age, and retinal ganglion cells (RGC) degenerate, usually starting at an age of approximately six months. In this chapter, we show how RGC degeneration in two-year-old DBA/2J mice has almost reached an end-point. We investigated visual function in these animals using electroretinography (ERG) and visual evoked potentials (VEP), and we checked the number of remaining RGC by retrograde staining. Almost no RGC were left in the retina, and VEP were hardly recordable. Surprisingly, also ERG amplitudes of scotopic a-waves and b-waves, photopic b-waves and oscillatory potentials were decreased significantly by approximately 40% compared to amplitudes measured in age-matched C57BL/6J mice. The latencies were not changed in DBA/2J

* Corresponding author: Peter Heiduschka, University of Münster Eye Hospital, Domagkstr. 15, D-48149 Münster, Germany; peter.heiduschka@ukmuenster.de; Tel: +49 251 83 57532; Fax: +49 251 83 5254959120.

mice compared to controls, and so were the ratios between amplitudes of a-waves, b-waves and oscillatory potentials. Our results indicate that, in addition to degeneration of RGC, also photoreceptors are affected by pathological processes in the eye caused by the mutations present in DBA/2J mice.

Keywords: DBA/2J, mice, retinal ganglion cells, electroretinography, visual evoked potentials, retrograde labelling, glaucoma

INTRODUCTION

Glaucoma is the second leading cause for blindness worldwide and affects approximately 3% of the population with a higher incidence at people aged 40 year and older (Krieglstein, 1993). Glaucoma represents a group of optic neuropathies characterised by the progressive loss of retinal ganglion cells (RGC) and their axons within the optic nerve (Quigley, 1999). Pigment dispersion glaucoma is one important form of glaucoma. In this disease, pigment particles that normally are located on the iris get loose and distribute inside the anterior chamber. If the pigment particles are deposited onto the trabecular meshwork, the chamber fluid drainage is blocked, and the intraocular pressure (IOP) elevates, which is a strong risk factor of glaucoma (Niyadurupola and Broadway, 2008).

The DBA/2J mouse is a widely used inbred strain in cardiovascular biology, neurobiology, and sensorineural research. John et al. (1998) reported that the DBA/2J mouse develops progressive eye abnormalities that closely mimic human pigment dispersion glaucoma. Pigment dispersion and iris atrophy were also observed in DBA/2J mice usually at an age of six to eight months (John et al., 1998; Libby et al., 2005). John et al. (1998) already stated the hypothesis that some of the deteriorated cells could be macrophages. In a recent study, we showedIt could be shown that pigmented cells detach only from the anterior side of the iris and migrate into the trabecular meshwork (Schraermeyer et al., 2009). We could identify these cells were identified as macrophages with phagocytosed melanosomes, but not as iris pigment epithelium (IPE) cells or iridal melanocytes as initially expected.

The defects observed in DBA/2J mice have their origin in recessive mutations in the *Gpnmb* and *Tyrp1* genes (John et al., 1998; Chang et al., 1999; Anderson et al., 2002, 2008). The incidence and the extent of iris atrophy in DBA/2J mice increase with age, and the iris atrophy is usually severe at the age of 18 months (John et al., 1998). The IOP increases significantly by six to nine months of age and decreases to control values in old animals (John et al., 1997; John et al., 1998). As a consequence of the glaucoma developing in DBA/2J mice, the nerve fibre layer becomes thinner, and the number of RGC is greatly depleted, accompanied by optic nerve atrophy and disorganisation (John et al., 1998).

There is a high phenotypic variability in glaucoma development in the DBA/2J mice (Libby et al., 2005; Schlamp et al., 2006; Scholz et al., 2008). Nevertheless, glaucoma develops in nearly all eyes, the disease follows a predictable progressive path, and the majority of mice suffer increase of IOP, loss of RGC and optic nerve atrophy by 22 months of age (Jakobs et al., 2005; Libby et al., 2005; Schlamp et al., 2006). This consistency in glaucoma development in DBA/2J mouse makes this strain a useful tool to study glaucoma (Schuettauf et al., 2002).

The progression of glaucoma and degeneration of RGC have been studied by several authors. Decrease of RGC number has been reported by Schuettauf et al. (2002, 2004), Anderson et al. (2005), Jakobs et al., (2005), Libby et al., (2005), Schlamp et al., (2006) and Zhong et al. (2007).

It is straightforward to expect that visual function of DBA/2J mice is impaired with progression of the disease. The clear-cut way to determine functional loss is to measure visual evoked potentials (VEP) in these animals, because VEP give the best idea about the presence, the state and the function of RGC and their axons in the optic nerve.

There are also several reports on the use of pattern electroretinography (pERG) to study RGC function in DBA/2J mice performed by the group led by Porciatti (Nagaraju et al., 2007; Saleh et al., 2007), and the authors found a considerable decrease of amplitudes with increasing age. Although the function of RGC is reflected only by pERG, Harazny et al. (2009) recently found decreased amplitudes in DBA/2J mice also by Ganzfeld ERG at ages up to approximately 300 days.

In this study, we examined two-year-old DBA/2J mice that can be considered a kind of "end point" regarding the degeneration process caused by the disease. Our aim was to evaluate the extent of RGC degeneration in such old DBA/2J mice. Regarding the reports on functional loss in aged DBA/2J mice, we were interested whether visual function on both retinal and cortical levels could still be recorded, and how large the difference to wild type mice would be. For this purpose, we performed ERG and VEP measurements in aged DBA/2J mice and age-matched C57BL/6J mice and labelled RGC retrogradely to quantify them.

MATERIAL AND METHODS

Animals

All mice were handled according to German animal protection laws. All experiments were conducted in accordance with the Association for Research in Vision and Ophthalmology. DBA/2J and C57BL/6J mice were obtained from the European distributor of Jackson Laboratories mice (Charles River Laboratories) and were bred here for a maximum of two generations. All mice were kept under specific pathogen-free conditions at room temperature in a 12 h light/12 h dark cycle. For the DBA/2J strain, a special fat chow containing 5.5% fat instead of 4.5% was provided ad libitum. Control eyes were collected from C57BL/6J mice that did not display any ocular abnormalities.

Visual Electrophysiology

General Procedure

Eight animals of each strain were used for visual electrophysiology examinations. Mice were dark adapted over a period of at least 24 hours. The cornea of the eyes of the anaesthetised animals was de-sensitised with a drop of Novesine (Novartis Ophthalmics). The upper eyelids were retracted slightly by a surgical silk thread. The animals were placed onto a heated platform (37°C) during the measurements to keep their body temperature constant. A gold wire ring electrode was placed into the mouth to serve as a reference electrode. A stainless steel needle electrode was inserted into the tail of the animals for grounding. The pupils were dilated with a drop of Tropicamide (Novartis Ophthalmics). All these manipulations were performed under dim red light, without bringing the animal into ambient light after dark adaptation. The red light was switched off after finishing all the stages of animal preparation. After an additional 5 minutes to allow the pupils to dilate, measurement was started using the commercial RetiPort32 device from Roland Consult Systems (Brandenburg, Germany).

Electroretinography

Animals were anaesthetised by an intraperitoneal injection of a mixture of ketamine and xylazine (120 mg/kg ketamine, 10 mg/kg xylazine). Gold wire ring electrodes placed on the corneas of both eyes served as working electrodes. Standard electroretinographic measurements were performed simultaneously on both eyes, with scotopic flash ERG at eight different light intensities from 0.0003 to 100 cd·s/m², an additional run for scotopic oscillatory potentials at 100 cd·s/m², photopic 30 Hz Flicker at 3 cd·s/m² after 10 minutes of light adaptation, and finally photopic flash ERG and photopic oscillatory potentials at 100 cd·s/m². The time of measurement was 160 ms, with 512 data points per measured waveform. The analogue filters of the ERG device were set to the frequency ranges of 0.5 to 200 Hz for both scotopic and photopic flash ERG, 50 to 500 Hz for oscillatory potentials and 10 to 50 Hz for 30 Hz Flicker. In addition, the waveforms of the oscillatory potentials were digitally filtered offline using a DSP filter included in the software of the ERG device (-15 dB for f<10 Hz). Amplitudes of a-waves were measured from the baseline to the bottom of the a-wave trough, whereas b-wave amplitudes were measured from the bottom of the a-wave trough to the peak of the b-wave.

Parameters of photoreceptor response were computed by using the well-known relationship by Hood and Birch (1994), based on the theory by Lamb and Pugh (1992):

$$P3_{(i,t)} = Rm_{P3} \cdot \left(1 - e^{-i \cdot S (t - t_d)^2}\right) \text{ for } t \geq td \qquad (1)$$

with i – stimulus intensity, t - time after flash onset, P3 - sum of individual photoreceptor responses, Rm_{P3} - saturated response, t_d - delay that allows for biochemical and other recording latencies, S - sensitivity parameter.

We approximated measured a- and b-wave amplitudes to the parameters $R_{max,1}$ and $R_{max,2}$ (maximal response amplitudes), $i_{50,1}$ and $i_{50,2}$ (half-saturating light intensities) and n,1 and n,2 - exponents describing the slope of the Hill function using the biphasic equation

$$R = R_{max,1} \frac{i^{n,1}}{i^{n,1} + i_{50,1}^{n,1}} + R_{max,2} \frac{i^{n,2}}{i^{n,2} + i_{50,2}^{n,2}} \qquad (2)$$

firstly introduced without the exponent n in the monophasic shape by Naka and Rushton (1966), with R - response amplitude and i – intensity of light stimulus.

The parameters for the equations (1) and (2) were computed using self-written non-linear least-square routines in Borland Pascal. The range of the

ERG waveform from the beginning of the a-wave leading edge to the first intrusion of the b-wave was used for the calculation, yielding between 10 and 15 data points. All six parameters of the Naka-Rushton equation (2) were left free during the calculation. Eight data points were used for the fit, according to the eight different light intensities used for stimulation.

Visual Evoked Potentials

Animals were anaesthetised with an intraperitoneal injection of a solution of chloral hydrate in physiologic saline (0.42 mg chloral hydrate/kg). A self-tapping stainless-steel screw with a shaft diameter of 1.12 mm and a length of 3.18 mm (Y-TX00-2, Small Parts, Inc., Miami Lakes, Florida) served as a measuring electrode and was inserted more than one week before the measurement through the skull into the left visual cortex (1.5 mm laterally to the midline, 1.5 mm anterior to the lambda), penetrating the cortex to approximately 1 mm. For the actual measurement, the skin was opened; the screw was cleaned of connecting tissue and blood and connected to the amplifier. Both eyes were stimulated for the measurement. Visual evoked potentials were recorded, with scotopic flash VEP at eight different light intensities ranging from 0.0003 to 100 cd·s/m², and photopic flash VEP at 100 cd·s/m² after 10 minutes of light adaptation. The time of measurement was 160 ms, with 512 data points per measured waveform, and frequency range of 0.5 to 200 Hz. After finishing the measurements, the wound was stitched and antibiotic ointment applied.

The averaged signals of DBA/2J mice and wild-type mice were compared with respect to both latency and amplitude.

Retrograde Labelling and Immunohistochemistry

RGC were labelled retrogradely by injecting a solution of Fluorogold (FG; Fluorochrome, LLC, Colorado) in PBS and 2% DMSO into each of the *superior colliculi*, approximately 20 μl on each side. One week after the injection, animals were enucleated, retinas prepared and fixed in 4% paraformaldehyde in 0.1 M PBS, pH 7.4. Digital images of areas of flat whole-mounts on black nitro-cellulose filter paper (Sartorius, Germany) were taken using a fluorescence microscope (Axioplan2, Zeiss, Germany). RGC were counted in the images.

For the neurofilament staining of the whole-mounts, retinas from DBA/2J and C57BL/6J mice were fixed for 3 days, washed in PBS and treated with

Proteinase K for 20 min at 37°C. The enzyme reaction was stopped by 3% H_2O_2 for 5 min, followed by three washing steps with PBS for 10 min. Blocking was performed with 2% BSA, 0.1% NaN_3 and 1% Triton X100 in PBS. Retinas were incubated in a 1:50 dilution of an anti-neurofilament antibody (R&D Systems, Germany) for 3 days at 4°C, then washed 5 times in PBS for 1 h, blocked again for 1h and incubated overnight at 4°C with an Cy3-conjugated donkey anti-goat antibody (Dianova, Germany; 1:500). Stained whole-mounts were embedded in FluorSave (Calbiochem, Germany) and inspected using a fluorescent microscope.

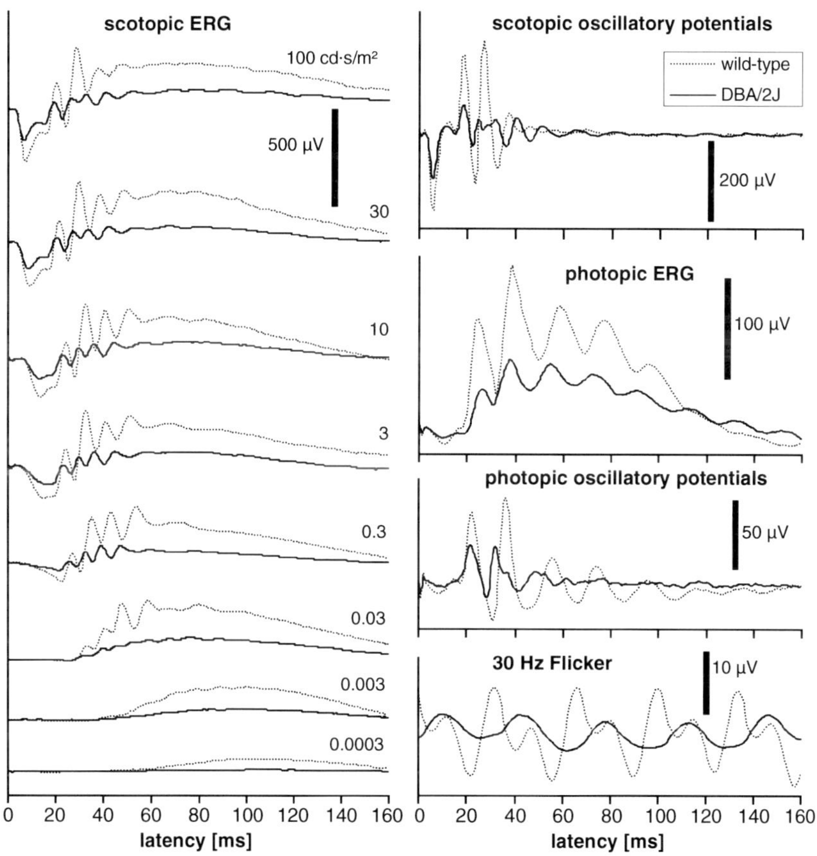

Figure 1. Representative appearance of electroretinographic waveforms obtained in wild-type C57BL/6J mice (dotted lines) and DBA/2J mice (solid lines). The intensities of light stimuli in scotopic ERG are indicated nearby the curves. Please note the different scales.

Statistics

The single ERG and VEP parameters as well as numbers of RGC obtained in DBA/2J mice and wild-type mice were compared using the Student's t-test.

RESULTS

Electroretinography

Typical examples of electroretinographic waveforms obtained in an aged DBA/2J mouse and an age-matched C57BL/6J mouse are shown in Figure 1. A clear impairment of retinal function in DBA/2J mice can be recognised at first sight; all waveforms of DBA/2J mice show considerably smaller amplitudes.

Results of numerical evaluation of the ERG parameters are shown in Figure 2. Amplitudes of a-waves are significantly smaller in DBA/2J mice at light intensities above 0.01 cd·s/m^2 ($p \leq 0.027$), and the same is true for the amplitudes of b-waves over the whole inspected range of light intensities ($p \leq 0.0018$) (Figure 2A). Based on the amplitude values, the Naka-Rushton parameters were calculated (Table 1). $R_{max,1}$ values are significantly smaller in DBA/2J mice than in C57BL/6J mice. $R_{max,2}$ values calculated for DBA/2J mice are also smaller, however, the difference to C57BL/6J mice $R_{max,2}$ values is not significant. No significant differences are present in all other parameters except for $i_{50,1}$ of b-wave amplitudes that is significantly smaller in C57BL/6J mice.

Parameters of equation (1) were calculated using the initial slope of the a-waves recorded in both mouse strains. The mean R_{max} value found in DBA/2J mice was significantly smaller than in C57BL/6J mice (-249 ± 52 µV vs. $--373 \pm 53$ µV, $p=0.0065$), whereas the sensitivity parameters S were quite similar in wild type mice and DBA/2J mice (0.00116 ± 0.00013 vs. 0.00123 ± 0.00026, $p=0.6210$).

The amplitudes of both scotopic and photopic oscillatory potentials (Figure 2B) and photopic b-waves (Figure 2C) are also significantly smaller in DBA/2J mice than in C57BL/6J mice. The ratio of the amplitudes of b-waves and a-waves, the so called b/a ratio, and the ratio of the amplitudes of oscillatory potentials and b-waves (OP/b ratio) were quite similar in both strains, although the values showed a higher variability in DBA/2J mice

(Figure 2D). There was also no significant difference in the OP/a ratio, although the value was slightly higher in DBA/2J mice, and the variability was much larger in DBA/2J mice (Figure 2D).

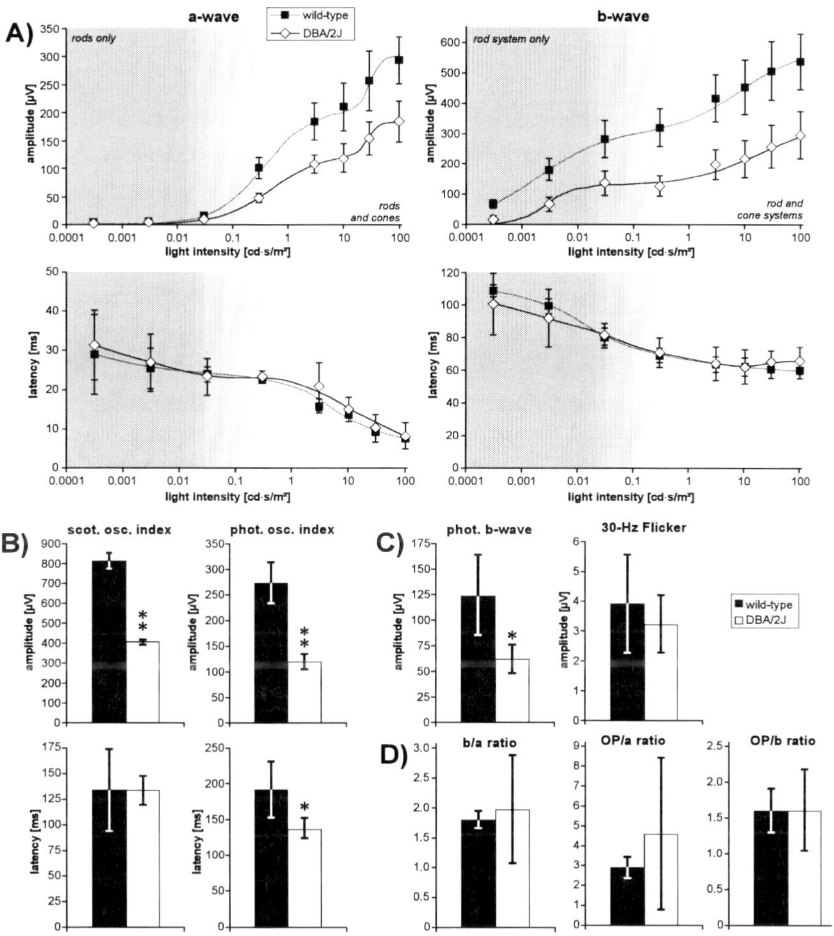

Figure 2. ERG parameters obtained in wild-type mice and DBA/2J mice. A) Amplitudes and latencies of scotopic ERG at different intensities of the light stimuli. The curves in the amplitude diagrams were calculated by the equation (2) using the parameters listed in table 1. The curves in the latency diagrams just serve to guide the eye and do not represent a function. B) Indices of amplitudes and latencies of scotopic and photopic oscillatory potentials. C) and D) Further parameters as indicated in the diagrams. The significance of parameter differences between wild-type mice and DBA/2J mice was indicated as follows: * $p<0.05$, ** $p<0.01$, *** $p<0.001$.

Table 1. Calculated parameters of the biphasic Naka-Rushton equation (2) with the amplitudes of electroretinographic a-waves and b-waves and VEP amplitudes. R_{max} values given in µV, n is without an dimension, and i_{50} values are given in cd·s/m²

	C57BL/6J n=8	DBA/2J n=8	p
ERG a-wave amplitudes			
$R_{max,1}$	207.7 ± 34.6	126.4 ± 19.7	0.0015
n,1	0.993 ± 0.155	0.926 ± 0.108	0.4639 (n.s.)
$i_{50,1}$	0.361 ± 0.183	0.486 ± 0.070	0.2127 (n.s.)
$R_{max,2}$	95.21 ± 30.65	58.38 ± 20.99	0.0597 (n.s.)
n,2	4.191 ± 2.732	4.534 ± 3.093	0.8567 (n.s.)
$i_{50,2}$	29.60 ± 11.29	27.05 ± 3.50	0.6651 (n.s.)
ERG b-wave amplitudes			
$R_{max,1}$	305.3 ± 69.2	129.1 ± 42.0	0.0009
n,1	0.729 ± 0.070	1.725 ± 1.156	0.0645 (n.s.)
$i_{50,1}$	0.0018 ± 0.0004	0.0027 ± 0.0006	0.0204
$R_{max,2}$	270.1 ± 84.8	205.9 ± 62.3	0.2184 (n.s.)
n,2	0.791 ± 0.268	0.709 ± 0.165	0.5936 (n.s.)
$i_{50,2}$	7.98 ± 4.58	17.18 ± 15.87	0.2144 (n.s.)
VEP amplitudes			
$R_{max,1}$	104.7 ± 28.3	10.9 ± 7.2	$6.77 \cdot 10^{-7}$
n,1	0.903 ± 0.275	1.025 ± 0.320	0.4925 (n.s.)
$i_{50,1}$	0.012 ± 0.005	0.009 ± 0.005	0.3540 (n.s.)
$R_{max,2}$	28.56 ± 17.28	3.86 ± 4.48	0.0026
n,2	3.199 ± 1.915	2.0 ± 0.6	0.1948 (n.s.)
$i_{50,2}$	7.12 ± 4.26	4.75 ± 2.34	0.2769 (n.s.)

There was no significant difference in the latencies of a-waves, b-waves and oscillatory potentials between DBA/2J mice and wild-type mice, except for the latency of photopic oscillations that were shorter in DBA/2J mice (Figures 2A and 2B).

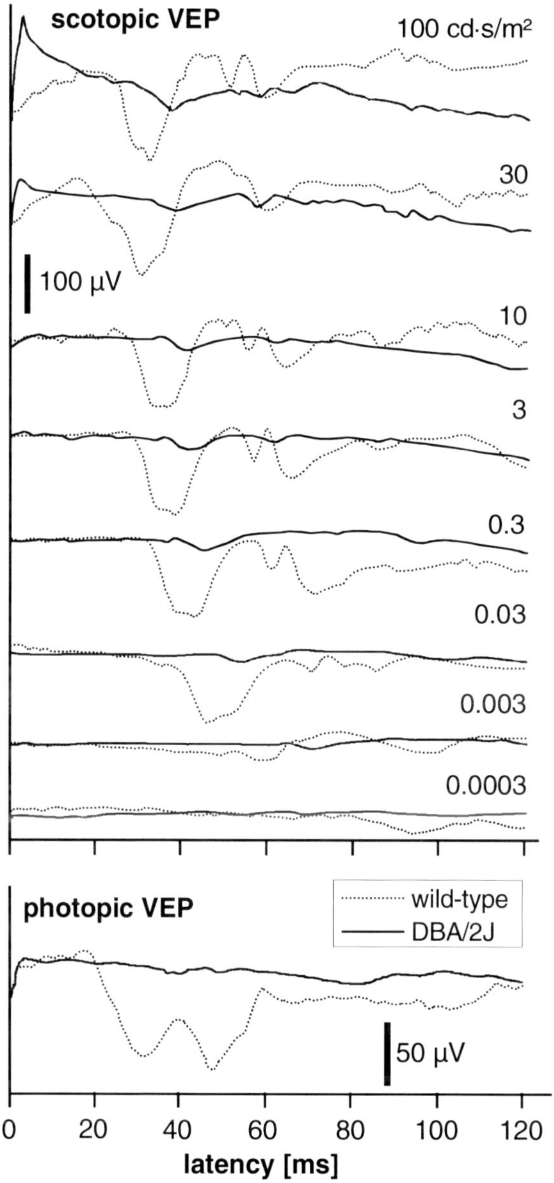

Figure 3. Typical appearance of waveforms of visual evoked potentials obtained in wild-type C57BL/6J mice (dotted lines) and DBA/2J mice (solid lines). The intensities of light stimuli in scotopic VEP are indicated nearby the curves. Please note the different scales.

Visual Evoked Potentials

Typical examples of VEP waveforms obtained in an aged DBA/2J mouse and an age-matched C57BL/6J mouse are shown in Figure 3. Almost no cortical activity can be recorded in DBA/2J mice upon light stimulation. Consequently, values of VEP amplitudes are significantly smaller in DBA/2J mice for both scotopic and photopic VEPs (Figure 4A). In some cases, it was difficult to determine the values of the VEP amplitudes at all due to the flat appearance of the waveforms. Therefore, we used a latency window ranging 30-40 ms around the latency obtained in C57BL/6J mice as a criterion whether a signal could be still interpreted as an evoked potential or if it was just a deflection due to spontaneous cortical activity.

The latencies measured in DBA/2J mice show a clear tendency of being prolonged compared to C57BL/6J mice, and the difference is significant at higher light intensities (Figure 4B). The variability of the latency values was higher in DBA/2J mice than in wild-type mice.

Comparison of Naka-Rushton parameters showed that the R_{max} values are significantly smaller in DBA/2J mice, whereas no significant differences were found in the other parameters (Table 1).

Numbers of Retinal Ganglion Cells

In DBA/2J mice, only a few RGC were left in the retina compared to age-matched C57BL/6J mice (Figure 5). Consequently, counting of RGC resulted in a significantly lower number of RGC in DBA/2J mice (3069 ± 350 RGC/mm² in C57BL/6J mice vs. 68 ± 11 RGC/mm² in DBA/2J mice, $p=6 \cdot 10^{-6}$).

We also performed double staining of retinal whole mounts using an antibody against neurofilament to counter-stain the RGC (Figure 6). Neurofilament immunoreactivity (IR) was found in the RGC somata and their axons as well as, to a lesser degree, in retinal blood vessels. In rare cases, more RGC were found to be labelled by Fluorogold than by the anti-neurofilament antibody. There has been almost no case in the C57BL/6J mice that an RGC displayed neurofilament IR without being labelled with Fluorogold, and we did not find such a case in DBA/2J mice.

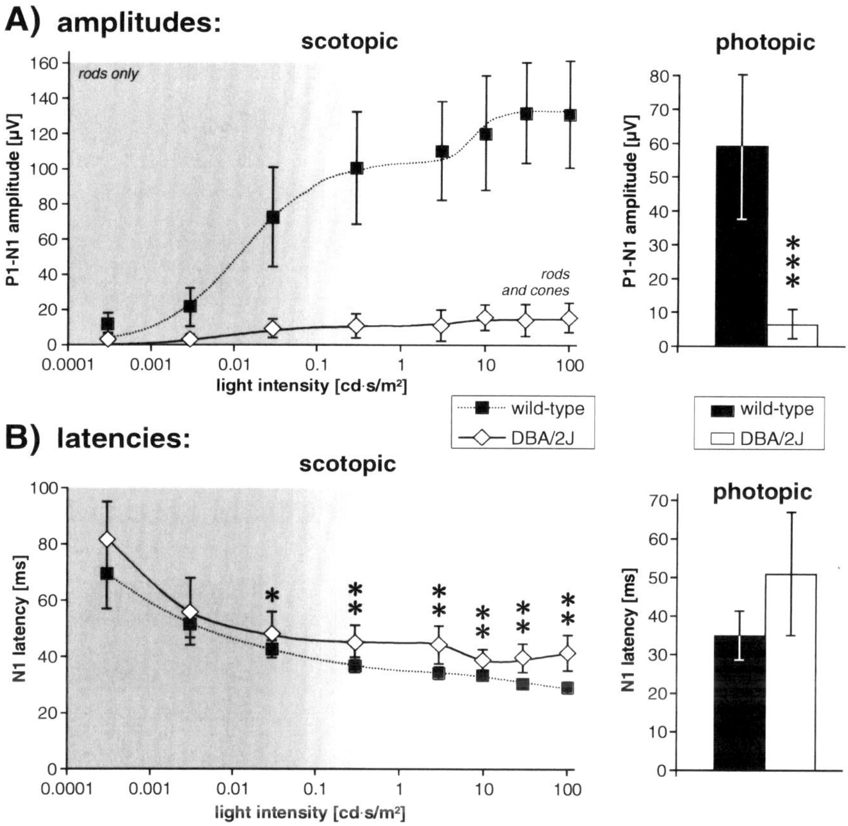

Figure 4. VEP parameters obtained in wild-type mice and DBA/2J mice. A) Amplitudes of scotopic VEP at different intensities of the light stimuli and of photopic VEP. The curves in the scotopic amplitude diagram were calculated by the equation (2) using the parameters listed in table 1. B) Latencies of scotopic VEP at different intensities of the light stimuli and of photopic VEP. The curves in the latency diagram just serve to guide the eye and do not represent a function. The significance of parameter differences between wild-type mice and DBA/2J mice was indicated as follows: * $p<0.05$, ** $p<0.01$, *** $p<0.001$.

Discussion

We examined the function of the retina and optic nerve in aged DBA/2J mice by ERG and VEP measurements. We found extremely reduced visual evoked potentials in the old DBA/2J mice. To our knowledge, it has been for the first time that VEP measurements have been performed in DBA/2J mice to check the function of the degenerated RGC and optic nerve. Moreover, ERG amplitudes were markedly decreased in DBA/2J mice.

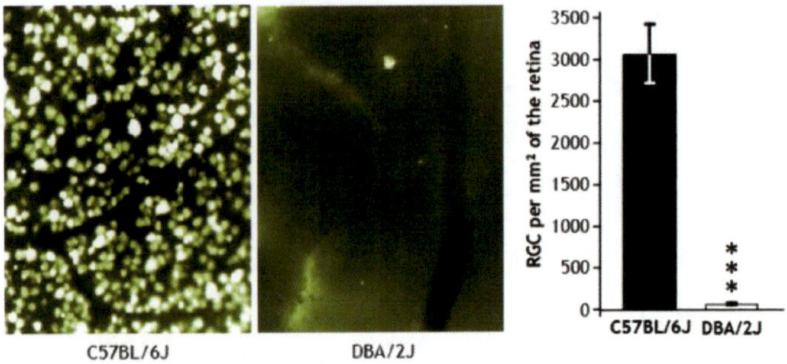

Figure 5. Representative fluorescence microscopy images of retinal whole mounts obtained from a C57BL/6J mouse and an age-matched DBA/2J mouse one week after retrograde staining of the RGC with Fluorogold. On the right side, a diagram shows the results of RGC counting in both animal models.

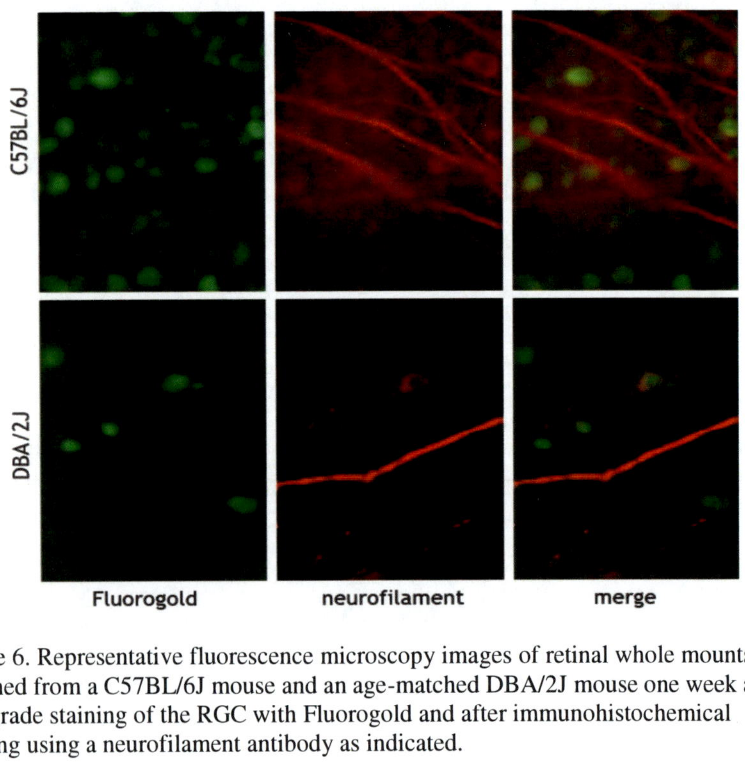

Figure 6. Representative fluorescence microscopy images of retinal whole mounts obtained from a C57BL/6J mouse and an age-matched DBA/2J mouse one week after retrograde staining of the RGC with Fluorogold and after immunohistochemical staining using a neurofilament antibody as indicated.

Finally, we checked the number of RGC by retrograde staining. We found a dramatically decreased number of RGC in retinal whole-mounts of aged DBA/2J mice, in an extent that the retina was almost devoid of RGC. Taking into account the continuous degeneration of RGC in the course of disease progression, such a result could be anticipated. Degeneration of RGC was quantified before in aged DBA/2NNia mice by retrograde staining, however, only until the age of 18 months (Danias et al., 2003). The authors found a by far higher number of surviving RGC than in our study, which may have its reason in the different DBA/2 strain they used. On the other hand, Jakobs et al. (2005) observed severe loss of RGC already in one-year-old DBA/2J mice by retrograde labelling, with large areas of the retina completely devoid of RGC.

According to the loss of RGC, VEP measurement revealed waveforms only hardly distinguishable from a flat line in some animals. Nevertheless, the decrease of the number of RGC in DBA/2J mice compared to C57BL/6J mice (Figure 5) is much higher in terms of percentage than the decrease of VEP amplitudes (Figure 4). It may be speculated that the remaining RGC give a higher input into the brain, be it by more intense action potentials and/or by a higher number of synapses the RGC axons form in their target area, possibly even with a higher number of neurons in the superior colliculus by forming additional axonal collaterals and sprouts in the target area. A similar finding, though in the case of RGC axons regenerating after an injury, was reported by Sauvé et al. (1995). It is possible that such a higher number of sprouts and synapses serve to compensate at least partially for the heavy loss of RGC. However, performing an analysis of neuronal circuits and synaptic density in the brain of DBA/2J mice was beyond the scope of this study.

ERG is a standard method to investigate retinal function, and pattern ERG (pERG) is applied to characterise the function of RGC. There are several reports on checking function of the RGC in DBA mice by pERG. Bayer et al. (2001a) measured pERG amplitudes in DBA/2NNia mice and C57BL/6 mice aged between two and ten months and found a decrease of amplitudes in DBA/2NNia mice compared to C57BL/6 mice, beginning at five to six months. Later on, pERG were measured in DBA/2J mice (Howell et al., 2007; Nagaraju et al., 2007; Saleh et al., 2007). Saleh et al. (2007) reported that the pERG amplitudes measured in DBA/2J mice were decreased by 50% at an age of eight months, although the retinal nerve fibre layer was still unaffected, and the pERG approached noise levels at an age of 11 months, although the retinal nerve fibre layer had lost only 40% of normal thickness. In contrast, we were able to detect at least some residual response when measuring VEP despite the almost complete degeneration of RGC in two-year-old DBA/2J mice.

Nagaraju et al. (2007) also reported on a decrease of pERG amplitudes 10-month-old DBA/2J mice, whereas photopic flash ERG amplitudes remained almost stable. In addition, artificial increase of IOP by tilting the mice into a head-down position caused a further decrease of pERG amplitudes, whereas a decrease of IOP by mannitol gave an increase in pERG amplitudes. Howell et al. (2007) demonstrated that RGC degeneration in DBA/2J mice could be delayed by the Wld^{s} mutation. Moreover, severe decline of pERG amplitudes could also be prevented.

Flash ERG measurements have been also performed in DBA mice, leading to different results. Bayer et al. (2001b) investigated the scotopic ERG response and retinal morphology in DBA/2NNia mice at ages between five and 15 months. They found a decrease of a-wave and b-wave amplitudes starting at an age of seven to eight months and progressing till the end of the study (15 months). Strikingly, the a-wave amplitude was found to decrease to almost zero at 15 months, in contrast to our findings in two-year-old mice.

Although the scotopic a-wave and b-wave amplitudes were also decreased significantly in our study, they still had considerable sizes indicating a partial activity of the photoreceptors and the retinal neurones. Nevertheless, the function of photoreceptors appears to be seriously disturbed in two-year-old DBA/2J mice. Although the b/a ratio values are almost the same in DBA/2J mice and C57BL/6J mice, it cannot be stated conclusively that the reduction of the b-wave amplitude is solely a direct consequence of the reduced input of the photoreceptors to bipolar cells and Müller cells, because the standard deviation of b/a ratio is very high in DBA/2J mice (Figure 2D).

Unfortunately, Bayer et al. (2001b) did not check photopic ERG in their animal model. Nagaraju et al. (2007) and Saleh et al. (2007) only checked photopic flash ERG amplitudes in the DBA/2J mouse and reported that they remained almost unchanged until an age of ten to eleven months, and they accounted this finding for a restriction of the degenerative processes to the RGC. Harazny et al. (2009) recently studied retinal function of DBA/2J mice in more detail by Ganzfeld flash ERG and reported on decreased scotopic a-wave and b-wave amplitudes as well as decreased amplitudes of oscillatory potentials and photopic Flicker ERG in DBA/2J mice at ages up to approximately 300 days. The reduced photopic Flicker ERG amplitudes reported by Harazny et al. (2009) may lead to the suggestion that they would probably have found also decreased photopic flash ERG b-wave amplitudes, if they would have tried this kind of measurement.

Bayer et al. (2001b) reported that the latencies of the a-wave remained almost the same compared to C57BL/6 mice, whereas latencies of b-waves were found to get longer with age. Such a prolongation of latencies was also reported by Harazny et al. (2009). This is in contrast to our results as we found an almost perfect match of the latencies of a-waves and b-waves. However, the evaluation of latencies depends strongly on the way they are determined. Bayer et al. (2001b) measured the time between the lowest point of the a-wave trough to the maximum of the subsequent incline of the waveform, and Harazny et al. (2009) took the time point of the stimulus as the start and the highest point of the oscillatory potentials as the end to determine the latency. In addition, Harazny et al. (2009) also used the highest point of the waveform after removal of the oscillation as the end point and called it the "corrected latency". In this case, latencies of DBA/2J mice and C57BL/6J mice were rather similar. This is in accordance to our results, as we always disregard the oscillations in the electroretinographic waveform when we determine amplitude and latency of the b-wave, and we also use the time point of the stimulus as a start.

Similar to Harazny et al. (2009), we also observed a decrease in the amplitudes of oscillatory potentials. The ratio between the amplitudes of the a-waves and the oscillatory potentials did not differ significantly between DBA/2J mice and C57BL/6J mice in our study. Again, there is a very high standard deviation in the OP/a ratio values in the DBA/2J mice. Together with the almost the same OP/b ratio values in both strains, it could be suggested that the neuronal circuitries of the inner retina are not harmed noticeably by the disease in the DBA/2J mice. The slightly increased average OP/a ratio value in DBA/2J mice could even lead to the speculation that the inner retina tries to compensate for the loss of input from the photoreceptors.

It is not straightforward to expect a decrease of flash ERG amplitudes in an animal model where primarily RGC are affected by the progressing disease. In a recent study, we also performed electrophysiological measurements in an animal model displaying RGC death with increasing age, the OPA1 mouse model (Alavi et al., 2007). Whereas there was a clear decrease in VEP amplitudes in the aged OPA1 mouse compared to age-matched wild-type mice, the ERG amplitudes and latencies were found to be almost the same (Heiduschka et al., 2010).

The finding of a decrease of a-wave amplitudes is a strong indication of an impairment of the function of photoreceptors and raises the question about structural integrity of photoreceptors. In several studies, no degeneration or other changes to the photoreceptors were reported (John et al., 1998; Schuettauf et al., 2004; Libby et al., 2005). Accordingly, Kendell et al. (1995) reported that they had not observed any photoreceptor loss in human glaucoma patients. In contrast, Nork et al. (2000) describe a swelling and a loss of photoreceptors in the eyes of glaucoma patients (red-green cones and rods) and a glaucoma model in monkeys.

In other studies performed in DBA/2J mice until the age of 18 months, we did not observe any irregularities in the photoreceptor layer (Schnichels et al., 2007; Schraermeyer et al., 2009). Future investigations will focus on even older retinas, as the reduction of a-wave amplitudes still requires an explanation.

As a summarising conclusion, we investigated visual function in two-year-old DBA/2J mice. There were only weak visual evoked potentials recordable, which was not surprising given the extremely low number of RGC found in the retina. However, also flash ERG amplitudes were decreased clearly. Whether only the function of photoreceptors is impaired or if there are also structural deficits in the photoreceptors of old DBA/2J mice, remains to be elucidated.

Financial Disclosure

Both authors disclose any commercial interest in the subject of the manuscript or in entities discussed in the manuscript.

References

Alavi, M.V., Bette, S., Schimpf, S., Schuettauf, F., Schraermeyer, U., Wehrl, H.F., Ruttiger, L., Beck, S.C., Tonagel, F., Pichler, B.J., Knipper, M., Peters, T., Laufs, J., Wissinger, B., 2007. A splice site mutation in the murine Opa1 gene features pathology of autosomal dominant optic atrophy. *Brain* 130, 1029-1042.

Anderson, M.G., Libby, R.T., Gould, D.B., Smith, R.S., John, S.W., 2005. High-dose radiation with bone marrow transfer prevents neurodegeneration in an inherited glaucoma. *Proc. Natl. Acad. Sci.* U.S.A. 102, 4566-4571.

Anderson, M.G., Nair, K.S., Amonoo, L.A., Mehalow, A., Trantow, C.M., Masli, S., John, S.W., 2008. GpnmbR150X allele must be present in bone marrow derived cells to mediate DBA/2J glaucoma. *BMC Genet.* 9, 30.

Anderson, M.G., Smith, R.S., Hawes, N.L., Zabaleta, A., Chang, B., Wiggs, J.L., John, S.W., 2002. Mutations in genes encoding melanosomal proteins cause pigmentary glaucoma in DBA/2J mice. *Nat. Genet. 30*, 81-85.

Bayer, A.U., Brodie, S.E., Mittag, T., 2001a. [Pilot study of pattern-electroretinographic changes in the DBA/2NNia mouse. Animal model of congenital angle-closure glaucoma]. O*phthalmologe* 98, 248-252.

Bayer, A.U., Neuhardt, T., May, A.C., Martus, P., Maag, K.P., Brodie, S., Lütjen-Drecoll, E., Podos, S.M., Mittag, T., 2001b. Retinal morphology and ERG response in the DBA/2NNia mouse model of angle-closure glaucoma. *Invest. Ophthalmol. Vis. Sci.* 42, 1258-1265.

Chang, B., Smith, R.S., Hawes, N.L., Anderson, M.G., Zabaleta, A., Savinova, O., Roderick, T.H., Heckenlively, J.R., Davisson, M.T., John, S.W., 1999. Interacting loci cause severe iris atrophy and glaucoma in DBA/2J mice. *Nat. Genet.* 21, 405-409.

Danias, J., Lee, K.C., Zamora, M.F., Chen, B., Shen, F., Filippopoulos, T., Su, Y., Goldblum, D., Podos, S.M., Mittag, T., 2003. Quantitative analysis of retinal ganglion cell (RGC) loss in aging DBA/2NNia glaucomatous mice: comparison with RGC loss in aging C57/BL6 mice. *Invest. Ophthalmol. Vis. Sci.* 44, 5151-5162.

Harazny, J., Scholz, M., Buder, T., Lausen, B., Kremers, J., 2009. Electrophysiological deficits in the retina of the DBA/2J mouse. *Doc. Ophthalmol.* 119, 181-197.

Heiduschka, P., Schnichels, S., Fuhrmann, N., Hofmeister, S., Schraermeyer, U., Wissinger, B., Alavi, M.V., 2010. Electrophysiological and histologic assessment of retinal ganglion cell fate in a mouse model for OPA1-associated autosomal dominant optic atrophy. *Invest. Ophthalmol. Vis. Sci.* 51, 1424-1431.

Hood, D.C., Birch, D.G., 1994. Rod phototransduction in retinitis pigmentosa: Estimation and interpretation of parameters derived from the rod a-wave. *Invest. Ophthalmol. Vis. Sci.* 35, 2948-2961

Howell, G.R., Libby, R.T., Jakobs, T.C., Smith, R.S., Phalan, F.C., Barter, J.W., Barbay, J.M., Marchant, J.K., Mahesh, N., Porciatti, V., Whitmore, A.V., Masland, R.H., John, S.W., 2007. Axons of retinal ganglion cells are insulted in the optic nerve early in DBA/2J glaucoma. *J. Cell. Biol.* 179, 1523-1537.

Jakobs, T.C., Libby, R.T., Ben, Y., John, S.W., Masland, R.H., 2005. Retinal ganglion cell degeneration is topological but not cell type specific in DBA/2J mice. *J. Cell. Biol.* 171, 313-325.

John, S.W., Hagaman, J.R., MacTaggart, T.E., Peng, L., Smithes, O., 1997. Intraocular pressure in inbred mouse strains. *Invest. Ophthalmol. Vis. Sci.* 38, 249-253.

John, S.W., Smith, R.S., Savinova, O.V., Hawes, N.L., Chang, B., Turnbull, D., Davisson, M., Roderick, T.H., Heckenlively, J.R., 1998. Essential iris atrophy, pigment dispersion, and glaucoma in DBA/2J mice. *Invest. Ophthalmol. Vis. Sci.* 39, 951-962.

Kendell, K.R., Quigley, H.A., Kerrigan, L.A., Pease, M.E., Quigley, E.N., 1995. Primary open-angle glaucoma is not associated with photoreceptor loss. *Invest. Ophthalmol. Vis. Sci.* 36, 200-205.

Krieglstein, G.K., 1993. [Blindness caused by glaucoma]. Ophthalmologe 90, 554-556.

Lamb, T.D., Pugh, E.N. Jr., 1992. A quantitative account of the activation steps involved in phototransduction in amphibian photoreceptors. *J. Physiol.* 499, 719-758

Libby, R.T., Anderson, M.G., Pang, I.H., Robinson, Z.H., Savinova, O.V., Cosma, I.M., Snow, A., Wilson, L.A., Smith, R.S., Clark, A.F., John, S.W., 2005. Inherited glaucoma in DBA/2J mice: pertinent disease features for studying the neurodegeneration. *Vis. Neurosci.* 22, 637-648.

Nagaraju, M., Saleh, M., Porciatti, V., 2007. IOP-dependent retinal ganglion cell dysfunction in glaucomatous DBA/2J mice. *Invest. Ophthalmol. Vis. Sci.* 48, 4573-4579.

Naka, K.I., Rushton, W.A., 1966. S-potentials from colour units in the retina of fish (Cyprinidae). J. Physiol. 185, 536-555.

Niyadurupola, N., Broadway, D.C., 2008. Pigment dispersion syndrome and pigmentary glaucoma - a major review. *Clin. Experiment. Ophthalmol.* 36, 868-882.

Nork, T.M., Ver Hoeve, J.N., Poulsen, G.L, Nickells, R.W., Davis, M.D., Weber, A.J., Vaegan, Sarks, S.H., Lemley, H.L., Millecchia, L.L., 2000. Swelling and loss of photoreceptors in chronic human and experimental glaucomas. *Arch. Ophthalmol.* 118, 235-245.

Quigley, H.A., 1999. Neuronal death in glaucoma. *Prog. Retin. Eye Res.* 18, 39-57.

Saleh, M., Nagaraju, M., Porciatti, V., 2007. Longitudinal evaluation of retinal ganglion cell function and IOP in the DBA/2J mouse model of glaucoma. Invest. *Ophthalmol. Vis. Sci.* 48, 4564-4572.

Sauvé, Y., Sawai, H., Rasminsky, M., 1995. Functional synaptic connections made by regenerated retinal ganglion cell axons in the superior colliculus of adult hamsters. *J. Neurosci.* 15, 665-675.

Schlamp, C.L., Li, Y., Dietz, J.A., Janssen, K.T., Nickells, R.W., 2006. Progressive ganglion cell loss and optic nerve degeneration in DBA/2J mice is variable and asymmetric. *BMC Neurosci.* 7, 66.

Schnichels, S., Conrad, S., Warstat, K., Henke-Fahle, S., Skutella, T., Schraermeyer, U., Julien, S., 2007. Gene expression of the repulsive guidance molecules/neogenin in the developing and mature mouse visual system: C57BL/6J vs. the glaucoma model DBA/2J. *Gene Expr. Patterns* 8, 1-11.

Scholz, M., Buder, T., Seeber, S., Adamek, E., Becker, C.M., Lütjen-Drecoll, E., 2008. Dependency of intraocular pressure elevation and glaucomatous changes in DBA/2J and DBA/2J-Rj mice. *Invest. Ophthalmol. Vis. Sci.* 49, 613-621.

Schraermeyer, M., Schnichels, S., Julien, S., Heiduschka, P., Bartz-Schmidt, K.U., Schraermeyer, U., 2009. Ultrastructural analysis of the pigment dispersion syndrome in DBA/2J mice. *Graefes Arch. Clin. Exp. Ophthalmol.* 247, 1493-1504.

Schuettauf, F., Quinto, K., Naskar, R., Zurakowski, D., 2002. Effects of anti-glaucoma medications on ganglion cell survival: the DBA/2J mouse model. *Vision Res.* 42, 2333-2337.

Schuettauf, F., Rejdak, R., Walski, M., Frontczak-Baniewicz, M., Voelker, M., Blatsios, G., Shinoda, K., Zagorski, Z., Zrenner, E., Grieb, P., 2004. Retinal neurodegeneration in the DBA/2J mouse-a model for ocular hypertension. *Acta Neuropathol.* 107, 352-358.

Zhong, L., Bradley, J., Schubert, W., Ahmed, E., Adamis, A.P., Shima, D.T., Robinson, G.S., Ng, Y.S., 2007. Erythropoietin promotes survival of retinal ganglion cells in DBA/2J glaucoma mice. *Invest. Ophthalmol. Vis. Sci.* 48, 1212-1218.

In: Ganglion Cells
Editor: Liora G. Vlastimil
ISBN: 978-1-63117-432-2

Chapter 4

WHAT HAVE WE LEARNED FROM CULTURED ADULT DORSAL ROOT GANGLION NEURONS?

***Kazunori Sango*[*1], *Naoko Niimi*[1], *Masami Tsukamoto*[1,2], *Kazunori Utsunomiya*[2], *Kunihiko Sakumi*[3], *Yusaku Nakabeppu*[3], *Toshihiko Kadoya*[4] and *Hidenori Horie*[5]**

[1] Laboratory of Peripheral Nerve Pathophysiology, Department of Sensory and Motor Systems, Tokyo Metropolitan Institute of Medical Science, Setagaya-ku, Tokyo, Japan

[2] Division of Diabetes, Metabolism & Endocrinology, Department of Internal Medicine, Jikei University School of Medicine, Minato-ku, Tokyo, Japan

[3] Division of Neurofunctional Genomics, Department of Immunobiology and Neuroscience, Medical Institute of Bioregulation, Kyushu University, Fukuoka, Japan

[4] Department of Biotechnology, Maebashi Institute of Technology, Maebashi, Gunma, Japan

[5] TechnoMaster Co., Ltd., Yokohama, Japan

[*] Address correspondence to: Kazunori Sango, MD, PhD; Laboratory of Peripheral Nerve Pathophysiology, Department of Sensory and Motor Systems, Tokyo Metropolitan Institute of Medical Science, 2-1-6 Kamikitazawa, Setagaya-ku, Tokyo 156-8506, Japan; Tel: 81-3-6834-2359, Fax: 81-3-5316-3150; E-mail: sango-kz@igakuken.or.jp.

ABSTRACT

Dorsal root ganglion (DRG) neurons are constituents of the peripheral sensory nervous system, and methods for their primary culture from embryonic, neonatal, and adult animals have been established. Because some biological properties of DRG neurons can change with maturation and aging, adult DRG neurons appear to be a better choice for studies on axonal regeneration after injury and peripheral neuropathies than immature neurons. In dissociated cell culture, each of the ganglion neurons is mechanically and enzymatically isolated and seeded in a substrate-coated culture dish. Because of the good yield of ganglion neurons with high purity and viability, various assays can be performed on these neurons (e.g., cell attachment, cell viability, neurite outgrowth activity, electrophysiology, and immunocytochemistry). In explant culture, ganglia associated with nerve fibers are embedded in a collagen gel or Matrigel, and the number and length of neurites outgrowing from nerve-transected terminals are measured. Because cell–cell interactions are maintained in an explanted tissue, it is likely that an explant culture system mimics nerve regeneration *in vivo* better than a dissociated cell culture system. Using these culture systems, we investigated mechanisms of action of several different molecules that regulate axonal regeneration (e.g., ciliary neurotrophic factor, galectin-1, exendin-4, and chondroitin sulfate proteoglycans). In addition, these culture methods have been applied to animal models of aging and diseases (e.g., diabetes, G_{M2} gangliosidosis, and systemic lupus erythematosus) to elucidate the pathogenesis of neurological disorders that result from those conditions.

Keywords: Dorsal root ganglion neurons, adult mice and rats, tissue culture, axonal regeneration, murine disease models

INTRODUCTION

Peripheral nerve regeneration with functional recovery after injury and the cure of various neuropathies have been anticipated, but have yet to be achieved by medical science. Recovery from peripheral nerve injury requires both neuronal cell survival and axonal regeneration across the site of injury and along the distal nerve stump as well as functional reconnection with the appropriate targets. There is no doubt that successful nerve regeneration depends on the intrinsic growth capacity coupled with an extracellular environment favorable for regeneration (Zochodne, 2008). A great number of molecules, such as neurotrophic factors and cytokines, cell adhesion molecules, and extracellular matrix components, have been implicated in the regenerative response to nerve injury (Terenghi, 1999), and therapeutic approaches using delivery systems for target genes have been receiving increasing attention (Mason et al., 2011). However, the signals that prompt neurons to extend processes in peripheral nerves after injury are not fully understood.

Tissue culture systems are useful for studies of peripheral nerve regeneration at the cellular level and allow researchers to investigate functional roles of various molecules in axonal regeneration. Dorsal root ganglion (DRG) neurons are constituents of the sensory system, and methods for their primary culture from embryonic, neonatal, and adult animals have been established (Peterson, 1999; Welch & Foster, 1999; Sango et al., 2006). Because of good neuronal yield in culture, various assays can be performed on DRG neurons (e.g., cell attachment, cell viability, neurite outgrowth activity, electrophysiology, and immunocytochemistry). Culture of neurons from peripheral ganglia other than DRG (e.g., vagal sensory neurons of jugular and nodose ganglia, sympathetic neurons of superior cervical ganglia, and parasympathetic neurons of ciliary and pterygopalatine ganglia) can also be performed on the basis of experimental animals (Moller et al., 1997; Saito et al., 2002), but the biological assays with these neurons are often limited by the low neuronal yield in culture. It is believed that some biological properties of the DRG neurons change with maturation and aging. For example, nerve growth factor (NGF) is essential for the survival of embryonic and neonatal DRG neurons, but not for the survival of adult neurons *in vitro* (Lindsay, 1988; Sango et al., 2008). During the postnatal period, a population of small DRG neurons initiate the expression of RET, the signal-transducing domain of the receptor for glial cell line-derived neurotrophic factor (GDNF), and downregulate the expression of TrkA, which is a high-affinity NGF receptor. With the emerging RET expression, these neurons switch from NGF dependence to dependence on GDNF (Molliver et al., 1997). In addition, some properties of DRG neural cell membranes, such as fluidity and elasticity, have been observed to decrease with age (Horie et al., 1986, 1990). Taking these age-related changes into account, it would be fair to say that the culture system of adult DRG neurons mimics peripheral nerve regeneration better than a culture system of immature neurons.

We applied the methods for dissociated cell culture and explant culture of DRG to adult rodents (Sango et al., 2006). In dissociated cell culture, each of the ganglion neurons is mechanically and enzymatically isolated and seeded in a substrate-coated culture dish. In explant culture, the ganglia associated with nerve fibers are embedded in a collagen gel (Figure 1). In this chapter, we address the advantages and disadvantages of these culture systems in relation to the research of axonal regeneration after injury and peripheral neuropathies. In addition, we review the previous and current studies on the 2 systems, primarily from our own laboratories.

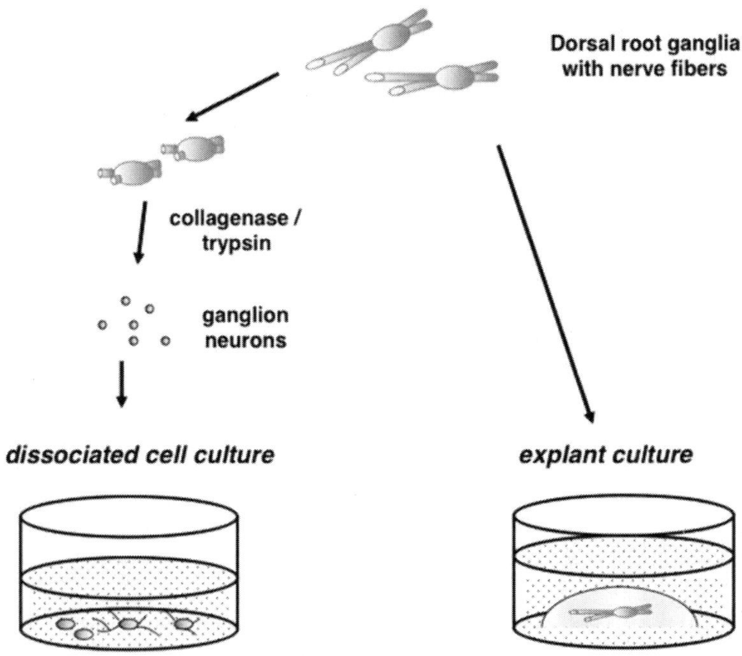

Figure 1. Schematic representation of the methods for dissociated cell culture and explant culture of neurons from dorsal root ganglia (DRG). In dissociated cell culture, each of the ganglion neurons is mechanically and enzymatically isolated and seeded in a culture dish precoated with extracellular substrate(s). In explant culture, DRG with nerve fibers are embedded in a collagen gel or Matrigel. The number and length of regenerating neurites from nerve-transected terminals are measured under a phase contrast microscope. [Reproduced with slight modifications from Sango et al., Curr. Diabetes Rev. (2006) 2:169–183, with permission from Bentham Science Publishers, Ltd.].

DISSOCIATED CELL CULTURE OF DRG NEURONS

Methods for primary culture of adult animal DRG neurons were developed by the end of the 1970s (Scott, 1977). However, in contrast to immature peripheral nervous system (PNS), the adult PNS contains a fully developed myelin sheath, epineurium, and perineurium, and therefore, compared with immature neurons, it is more time-consuming to obtain the adult neurons with high purity. Goldenberg and De Boni (1983) reported that density gradient centrifugation with Percoll increased the neuronal yield and eliminated most of the myelin sheaths and non-neuronal cells (e.g., Schwann cells, satellite cells, fibroblasts, and perineurial cells). Following this protocol with slight modifications, we can obtain more than 5×10^4 neurons together with a smaller number of non-neuronal cells per animal. DRG neurons are easily distinguished from non-neuronal cells by their larger cell size with round phase-bright cell bodies (Figure 2). The neuron-enriched DRG culture is subsequently prepared for Western blotting. In a typical experiment, we can excise almost 120 ganglia from the cervical to sacral levels from 3 mice, and dissociated neurons from these ganglia are subsequently seeded at high density ($>5 \times 10^3/cm^2$) in a 12-well tissue culture plate (Sango et al., 2007; Takaku et al., 2013).

Using the cell culture system, we investigated the mechanisms of how intrinsic and extrinsic factors alter neuronal viability and neurite outgrowth activity.

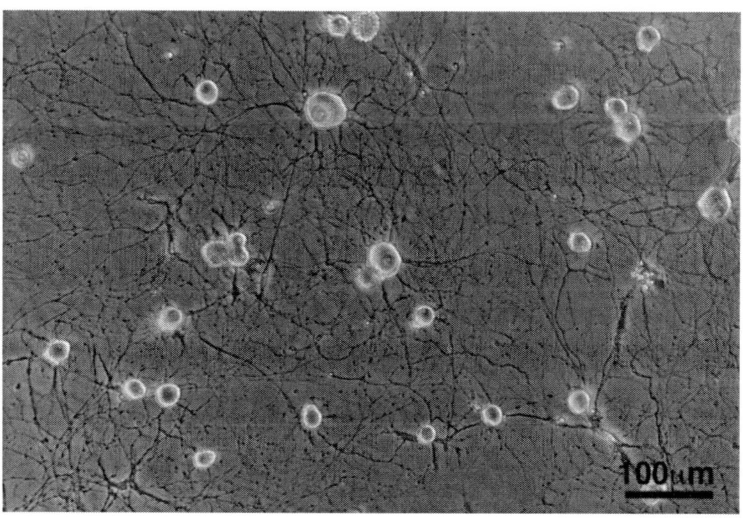

Figure 2. A phase contrast micrograph of adult rat DRG neurons after 4 days in culture.

EXPLANT CULTURE OF DRG

Although the dissociated cell culture of DRG neurons is useful for studying axonal regeneration, it has the following disadvantages:

I. Neurites are emerging from the surface of DRG neurons in the dissociated cell culture, while axonal regeneration *in vivo* occurs at the sites of injury.
II. Because DRG neurons are isolated from other neurons and non-neuronal cells during the dissociation procedure, we are unable to investigate cell–cell interactions that appear to play a key role in axonal regeneration *in vivo*.
III. We cannot rule out the possibility that severely injured neurons (e.g., from animals used as a disease model or neurons after exposure to toxic substances) are eliminated during the dissociation procedure and/or at the initial stage of culture, and the surviving neurons may be capable of extending neurites at the same rate as controls.

To resolve these problems, we established a 3-dimensional collagen gel culture system for DRG explants, in which adult DRG with nerve fibers are embedded in a collagen gel or Matrigel, and the number and length of regenerating neurites from nerve-transected terminals are measured under a phase contrast microscope by moving the focus point (Horie et al., 1991a; Figure 3). Because the cell–cell interactions are maintained in the explanted tissues, it is reasonable to assume that the explant culture system mimics nerve regeneration *in vivo* better than the dissociated cell culture system. Using this culture system, we showed that various neurotrophic factors, cytokines, and co-cultured tissues can enhance neurite regeneration (Horie & Kadoya, 2000; Sango et al., 2006). These models may also be suitable for the evaluation of the effect of experimental diabetes on nerve regeneration *in vitro* (Sango et al., 2002a). It must be noted that the explant culture lacks the process of Wallerian degeneration, but can mimic the neural regenerative activity in the site proximal to injury. Therefore, the state of enhanced neurite outgrowth in explant culture does not necessarily indicate acceleration of functional recovery after axonal injury; rather, the excess of regenerating fibers may impair proper target reinnervation and subsequent functional repair (Yasuda et al., 2002). When some molecules or conditions exhibit neurite outgrowth-promoting activities in explant culture, it is necessary to confirm their efficacy for axonal regeneration in *in vivo* experiments.

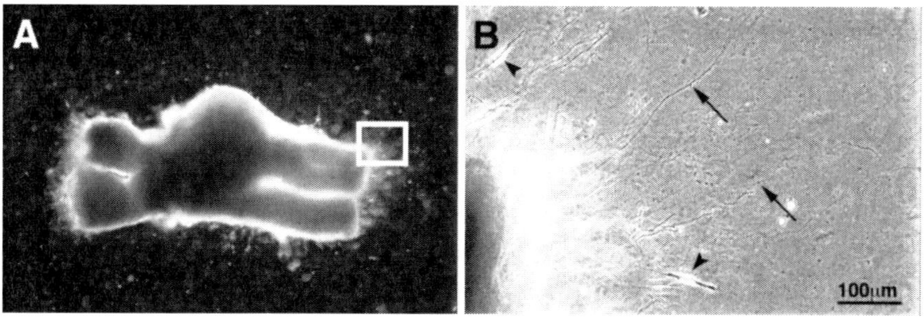

Figure 3. Explant culture of adult rat DRG. (A) DRG with spinal nerve bundles embedded in Matrigel. (B) A phase contrast micrograph of regenerating neurites (arrows) and migrating Schwann cells (arrowheads) from a transected nerve site (the same region enclosed by the white rectangle in panel A). [Reproduced from Sango et al., Histochem. Cell Biol. (2007) 128:35–43, with permission from Springer].

FACTORS INVOVLVED IN AXONAL REGENERATION

Ciliary Neurotrophic Factor (CNTF)

CNTF is a member of the interleukin-6 cytokine family, which includes leukemia inhibitory factor (LIF), interleukins 6 and 11 (IL-6 and IL-11), oncostatin M (OSM), cardiotrophin 1 (CT-1), cardiotrophin-like cytokine (CLC), and neuropoietin (Sendtner et al., 1994; Halvorsen & Kaur, 2006). All the family members utilize the receptor subunit gp130 to initiate signal transmission (Zigmond, 2012). CNTF acts on neurons through several cell surface receptors [i.e., CNTF receptor α (CNTFR-α), gp130, and LIF receptor (LIFR)]: (1) The binding of CNTF to CNTFR-α triggers heterodimerization of gp130 and LIFR, which form an active trimeric receptor complex in the plasma membrane (Davis et al., 1993). (2) The receptor complex activates the Janus family of tyrosine kinases (Jak1/Jak2), thereby leading to tyrosine phosphorylation, dimerization, and nuclear translocation of signal transducer and transcription activator (STAT; primarily STAT3). (3) The phosphorylated STAT3 dimers bind to specific DNA response elements in promoter regions to activate transcription of target genes (Taga & Kishimoto, 1997). This Jak–STAT signaling pathway is likely to play a major role in the neuropoietic function of CNTF, although receptor-mediated retrograde axonal transport of this molecule to the neuronal cell bodies has also been suggested (Curtis et al., 1993). We observed that recombinant CNTF enhances survival and neurite outgrowth of cultured adult rat DRG neurons (Sango et al., 2008) and neurite outgrowth from DRG explants (Shuto et al., 2001). Among other neurotrophic factors (NGF and GDNF) and IL-6 family members (IL-6, LIF, CT-1, and OSM) at the same concentration (50 ng/mL), CNTF as well as LIF and OSM exhibited a strong capacity for the promotion of the percentage of viable neurons and neurite-bearing cells (Table 1). NGF and GDNF are known to be potent inducers of neurite elongation, although these molecules are less effective than CNTF at improving neuronal survival. CNTF enhances the proportion of neurite-bearing cells in both small (soma diameter, <30 μm) and large neurons (soma diameter, ≥30 μm), whereas NGF and GDNF boost the number of neurite-bearing cells, primarily among small neurons. These findings suggest that CNTF stimulates a wider subpopulation of DRG neurons than NGF and GDNF. Western blotting revealed that CNTF induces phosphorylation of STAT3, serine–threonine kinase Akt, and extracellular signal–regulated kinase (ERK) 1/2 in the neurons. Furthermore, the neurite outgrowth-promoting activity of CNTF is reduced by co-treatment with JAK2 inhibitor AG490, STAT3 inhibitor STA-21, phosphatidylinositol 3′-kinase (PI3K) inhibitor LY294002, and mitogen-activated protein kinase (MEK) inhibitor PD98059 in a concentration-dependent manner. The survival-promoting activity of CNTF is also affected by AG490, STA-21, and LY294002 at higher concentrations but not by PD98059.

These findings are suggestive of the involvement of the JAK2/STAT3, PI3K/Akt, and MEK/ERK signaling pathways in CNTF-induced neurite outgrowth, where the first 2 pathways are believed to play a major role in the survival response of neurons to CNTF (Sango et al., 2008; Figure 4). Through the gp130-mediated signaling pathways, CNTF and other IL-6-type cytokines have been shown to upregulate several relevant genes (Zigmond, 2012). In particular, the STAT3 and PI3K pathways operate sequentially to induce the expression of regeneration gene protein 2 (Reg-2), a member of the regenerating gene family in embryonic motoneurons (Nishimune et al., 2000). Reg-2 is not expressed in intact DRG, but is rapidly upregulated after sciatic nerve injury (Averill et al., 2002) and adjuvant-induced monoarthritis (Averill et al., 2008). In our preliminary study, treatment with CNTF for 24 h induced the expression of Reg-2 in the nuclei of DRG neurons (arrows in Figure 5). Although further research is required, Reg-2 appears to be a downstream target molecule of CNTF, and Reg-2 plays a neuroprotective role in PNS after injury. Similarly, Fang et al. (2011) reported that intrathecal administration of Reg-2 significantly reduces neuronal death and inflammation in a rodent model of spinal cord transection injury.

Table 1. The relative effect of each recombinant protein on the survival and neurite outgrowth of cultured adult rat DRG neurons. Among these 7 molecules, CNTF exerted the highest activity on the survival ratios and proportions of neurite-bearing cells. NGF and GDNF were potent inducers of neurite elongation, though less effective than CNTF for neuronal survival. The IL-6 cytokines, except IL-6, enhanced both neuronal survival and neurite outgrowth

	Survival	Neurite outgrowth	
		Neurite-bearing cells	Neurite length
CNTF	++	++	+
NGF	± ~+	+	++
GDNF	-	+	++
IL-6	± ~+	-	-
LIF	++	++	+
CT-1	+~++	+	+
OSM	++	++	+

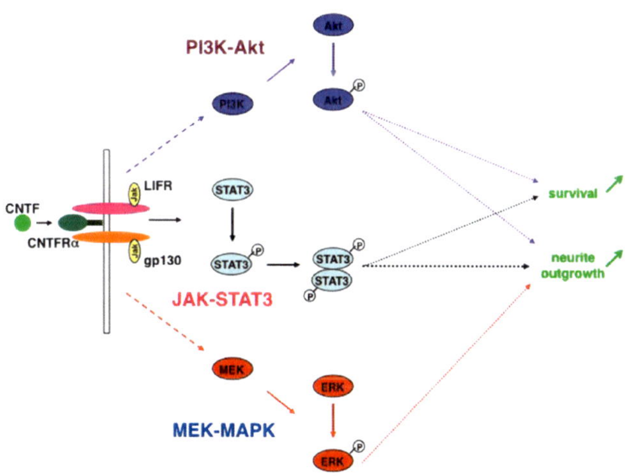

Figure 4. Possible signaling pathways mediating the effects of CNTF on cultured DRG neurons. The JAK-STAT3, PI3K-Akt, and MEK/ERK signaling pathways are involved in the CNTF-induced neurite outgrowth, whereas the JAK-STAT3 and PI3K-Akt pathways may play a major role in the survival response of neurons to CNTF.

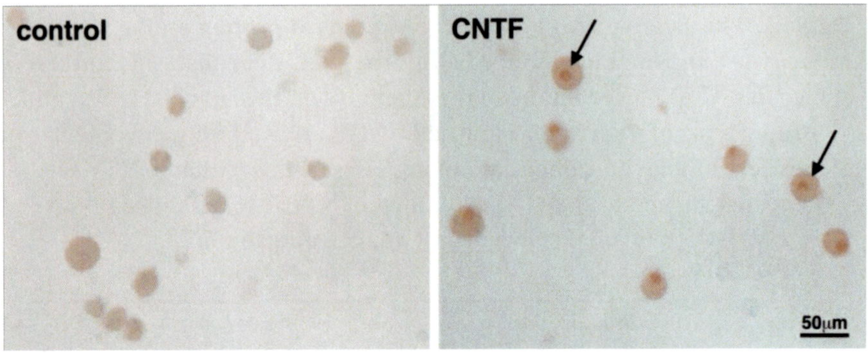

Figure 5. Immunocytochemical analysis with an anti-Reg-2 antibody. Treatment with 50 ng/mL of recombinant CNTF for 24 h induced expression of Reg-2 in the nuclei of adult rat DRG neurons (arrows).

Galectin-1 (GAL-1)

GAL-1, a member of the β-galactoside-binding animal lectin family, is believed to play a role in the development, degeneration, and regeneration of the nervous system (Camby et al., 2006; Sango et al., 2012a; Starossom et al., 2012). Despite lacking a leading signal peptide, GAL-1 is subject to secretion through the non-classical pathway from various types of cells, including DRG neurons and Schwann cells (Cooper & Barondes, 1990; Sango et al., 2004). After exiting the cell, some GAL-1 molecules associate with surface or extracellular matrix glycoconjugates, where the lectin activity is stabilized, whereas free GAL-1 molecules are rapidly oxidized in the non-reducing extracellular environment. Growing evidence suggests that both the reduced and oxidized forms of GAL-1 are involved in the repair process after nerve injury (Camby et al., 2006). However, there is a marked difference in the structural and functional properties between the two forms: GAL-1 in the reduced form acts on neural tissue as a lectin (Sasaki et al., 2004; Plachta et al., 2007), whereas GAL-1/Ox lacks the lectin activity, but acts as a cytokine-like molecule to promote axonal regeneration and Schwann cell migration through the stimulation of macrophages (Horie et al., 1999, 2004; Echigo et al., 2010; Sango et al., 2012).

Our immunohistochemical analysis revealed that GAL-1 is predominantly expressed in isolectin B4 (IB4)-binding small non-peptidergic (GDNF-responsive) neurons in the sections of adult rat DRG (Sango et al., 2012). In addition, both recombinant NGF and GDNF (50 ng/mL) stimulate neurite outgrowth in cultured adult rat DRG neurons, whereas GDNF, but not NGF, significantly increases the number of IB4-binding neurons and the relative protein expression of GAL-1 in the neuron-enriched culture of DRG. In our experiments, the GDNF-induced neurite outgrowth and GAL-1 upregulation are attenuated by an anti-RET antibody and PI3K inhibitor LY294002, suggesting that the neurite outgrowth-promoting activity of GDNF may be attributable, at least partially, to the upregulation of GAL-1 through the RET–PI3K pathway.

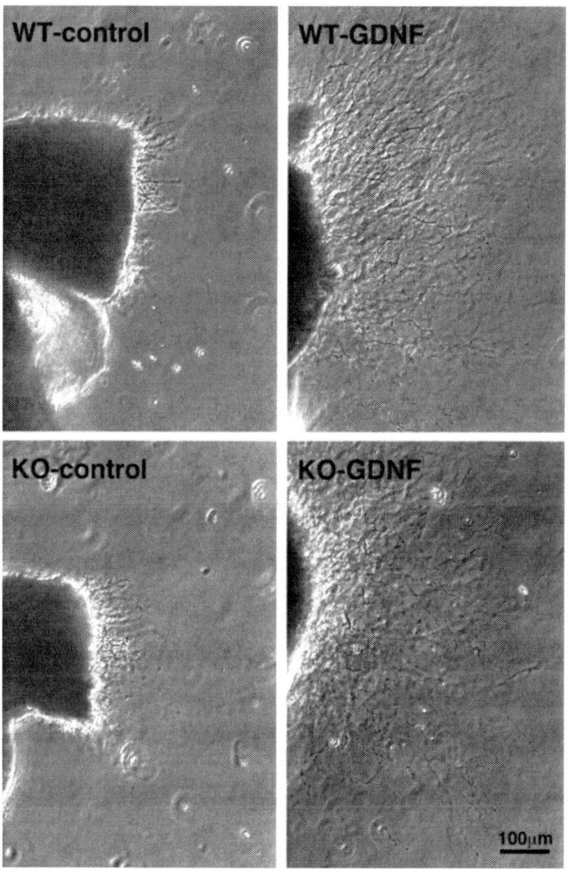

Figure 6. Phase contrast micrographs of regenerating neurites from transected nerve terminals of DRG explants from GAL-1 knockout (KO) and wild-type (WT) mice after 3 days in culture. The explants were maintained in a serum-free medium in the presence or absence (control) of GDNF (50 ng/mL).

In contrast, no significant differences were observed between GAL-1 knockout and wild-type mice in GDNF-induced neurite outgrowth in cultured DRG neurons and explants (Figure 6). Because a growing body of evidence indicates that GDNF promotes axonal regeneration after injury and regulates the sensitivity of thermal nociceptors, GAL-1 may play a major role in these phenomena, but the findings from GAL-1 knockout mice imply functional redundancy between GAL-1 and the other molecules. Furthermore, considerable immunohistochemical colocalization of GAL-3 with GAL-1 in DRG sections (Regan et al., 1986; Takaku et al., 2013) and GDNF-induced upregulation of both GAL-1 and GAL-3 in cultured DRG neurons (Takaku et al., 2013) allow us to assume redundancy of these galectins.

Exendin-4 (EX-4)

Glucagon-like peptide 1 (GLP-1) exhibits insulinotropic properties by stimulating specific G protein-linked receptors (GLP-1R) on pancreatic β cells in response to nutrient ingestion (Campbell & Drucker, 2013). GLP-1R is observed not only in the pancreas but also in extrapancreatic tissues, including the central and peripheral nervous systems (Harkavyi & Whitton, 2010). Recent studies are suggestive of the beneficial effects of GLP-1 on neurodegenerative disorders, such as Alzheimer's disease (McClean et al., 2011), Parkinson disease (Li et al., 2009), and peripheral neuropathies (Perry et al., 2007; Liu et al., 2011; Kan et al., 2012). Exendin-4 (Ex-4), a 39-amino acid peptide, shows bioactivities almost identical to those of GLP-1 and a substantially longer plasma half-life. Ex-4 reverses the neurological abnormalities of streptozotocin (STZ)-induced diabetic mice without normalizing blood glucose levels (Himeno et al., 2011); these data are suggestive of its direct action on PNS. We observed that GLP-1R is expressed in subpopulations of adult rat DRG neurons *in vivo* and *in vitro* and that Ex-4 dose-dependently (1 nM < 10 nM < 100 nM) promotes neurite outgrowth in adult rat DRG neurons after 2 days of culture (Sango et al., Neurodiab Congress, Barcelona, 2013). These findings imply potential efficacy of Ex-4 in the treatment of diabetic and other peripheral neuropathies. Our current work focuses on the signaling molecules and pathways activated by Ex-4 in DRG neurons.

Chondroitin Sulfate Proteoglycans (CS-PGs)

CS-PGs present in PNS are likely to participate in the process of axonal degeneration and regeneration as regulatory molecules in a manner similar to the processes occurring in the central nervous system (Cafferty et al., 2008). Most studies using sciatic nerve injury models (i.e., axotomy, crush, and entrapment) have demonstrated the upregulation of CS-PGs in the nerve tissue distal to the injury and inhibitory action of CS-PGs on axonal regeneration (Zuo et al., 1998). Consistent with the findings of *in vivo* studies, both endogenous and exogenous CS-PGs inhibit the adhesion and neurite outgrowth of DRG neurons (from immature and adult animals) in culture. Ferguson and Muir (2000) employed cryoculture assays, in which neonatal and adult mouse DRG neurons were grown on a substratum of sciatic nerve sections (unfixed) of an adult rat. Neurite outgrowth from these neurons was increased by pretreatment of the sections with chondroitinase ABC (ChABC) or matrix metalloproteinases (MMP-2 and MMP-9). Because ChABC and MMPs have been shown to degrade and inactivate CS-PGs, these findings suggest that endogenous CS-PGs are the primary inhibitors of peripheral nerve regeneration. Kuffler et al. (2009) reported inhibitory effects of CS-PGs from satellite Schwann cells on neurite outgrowth of adult human DRG neurons. Neurons free of soma contact with satellite cells or in soma contact with ChABC-treated satellite cells extended considerably longer neurites than neurons in soma contact with untreated satellite cells.

We tested the effects of exogenously applied CS-PGs on the biophysical properties of cultured adult rat DRG neurons (Sango et al., 2003, 2007). Phosphacan and neurocan used as coating substrata (1–10 μg/mL) significantly inhibit the adhesion and neurite outgrowth of DRG neurons. Treatment with these CS-PGs abrogates the positive effects of laminin and fibronectin on attachment and neurite outgrowth. These inhibitory effects are attenuated by the pretreatment of CS-PGs with ChABC. According to these findings, phosphacan and neurocan are repulsive substrata for adhesion and neurite outgrowth of cultured adult rat DRG neurons. Both CS chains and core proteins appear to be responsible for the inhibitory properties of these CS-PGs. In contrast, there is a possibility that CS-PGs, unlike simple barrier molecules, may be involved in the protection of neurons from cell death, in prevention of excess fiber regeneration, and in proper guidance of target reinnervation after axonal injury.

DRG Neurons from the Murine Models of Aging and Diseases

In addition to healthy adult rodents, we and others applied the methods of cell and explant culture of DRG to aged mice and murine models of diabetes, lysosomal storage diseases, and autoimmune diseases. Because culture of DRG neurons from experimental diabetic animals has been discussed in detail in other publications (Sango et al., 1997, 2006; Chowdhury et al., 2013), there is no need to dwell on this topic in this chapter.

Aged Mice

Dissociated neurons from DRG of aged mice (>24 months of age) exhibit deterioration of some plasma membrane functions, such as cell volume autoregulatory function under hypotonic conditions (Horie et al., 1989, 1993), membrane elasticity (Horie et al., 1990), and adhesion to type IV collagen and fibronectin (Sango et al., 1993) compared with young adult mice (3 months of age). In addition, the number and length of neurites regenerating from transected nerve terminals of DRG explants decreases with age of the mice. NGF promotes neurite outgrowth in both young adult and aged mice (Horie et al., 1991a). In agreement with this finding, a large population of DRG neurons from aged mice is responsive to NGF and acetyl-L-carnitine (Manfridi et al., 1992); NGF, but not acetyl-L-carnitine, increases the initial rate of neurite regeneration, whereas both NGF and acetyl-L-carnitine promote neuronal survival.

G_{M2} Gangliosidosis (Sandhoff Disease)

Sandhoff disease is an autosomal recessive hereditary neurodegenerative disorder, characterized by a deficient activity of lysosomal β-hexosaminidase and subsequent accumulation of the G_{M2} ganglioside and related glycolipids throughout the nervous system. Murine models of Sandhoff disease created by targeted gene disruption exhibit progressive manifestation of neurological problems starting approximately 3 months after birth as well as excessive glycolipid storage throughout the central nervous system and PNS (Sango et al., 1995; Phaneuf et al., 1996). Immunoelectron microscopic studies revealed conspicuous involvement of multilamellar inclusion bodies immunoreactive for the G_{M2} ganglioside in the cytoplasm of DRG neurons of mice with Sandhoff disease. We observed impaired neuronal survival in mice with Sandhoff disease, but the surviving Sandhoff neurons extend neurites to almost the same level compared with healthy mouse neurons (Sango et al., 2002b). In addition, some Sandhoff neurons survive longer than a month in culture. Therefore, lysosomal storage is unlikely to impair viability and neurite outgrowth of all DRG neurons. In a similar manner, cultured Schwann cells from mice with Sandhoff disease display lysosomal storage but survive and proliferate in culture (Sango et al., 2002b). We established immortalized Schwann cell lines from the long-term and Schwann cell-enriched culture (Ohsawa et al., 2005).

Systemic Lupus Erythematosus (SLE)

SLE is a multisystem autoimmune disease frequently complicated with nervous system damage. MRL-lpr/lpr mice spontaneously develop an autoimmune disease and lesions that are similar to those in human SLE (Cohen & Eisenberg, 1991) and appear to be useful for studies of the cross talk between the immune and nervous system. Hikawa et al. (1997) reported an age-related decrease in neurite outgrowth of DRG neurons from MRL-lpr/lpr mice (4–6 weeks > 16–20 weeks > 23–25 weeks). Those authors also reported an age-related increase of serum immunoglobulin G (IgG) levels in MRL-lpr/lpr mice, a finding, which suggests that the immunological dysfunction in this autoimmune disease is likely to affect axonal regeneration.

DRG Neurons Co-Cultured with Non-Neuronal Cells

Schwann Cells

Co-culture of Schwann cells and DRG neurons has been utilized as an experimental model to elucidate the mechanisms of neuron–Schwann cell interplay and myelination during development and regeneration of PNS (Kleitman et al., 1998). In most of the previously reported co-culture systems, however, both DRG neurons and Schwann cells have been derived from embryonic or neonatal animals (Päiväläinen et al., 2008; Xiao et al., 2009). We established spontaneously immortalized Schwann cell lines using long-term culture of adult Fischer 344 rat DRG and peripheral nerves. One of the cell lines, designated IFRS1 (immortalized Fischer rat Schwann cells 1), retained the distinct Schwann cell phenotype, namely spindle-shaped morphology with immunoreactivity for glial cell markers (e.g., S100, low-affinity NGF receptor p75, and GFAP). Light and electron microscopic analyses revealed that IFRS1 cells are capable of myelinating neurites in co-culture with adult rat DRG neurons (Sango et al., 2011). These data indicate that IFRS1 cells possess biological features of mature Schwann cells and are useful for the study of neuron–Schwann cell interactions in peripheral nerve degeneration and regeneration. Our current work with the DRG neuron–IFRS1 co-culture system is aimed to evaluate the efficacy of Ex-4 in axonal regeneration and remyelination (Sango et al., Neurodiab Congress, Barcelona, 2013).

Hepatocytes

Dissociated hepatocytes from adult mice, when co-cultured with DRG explants from adult and aged mice, significantly enhance neurite regeneration and neuronal survival (Horie et al., 1991b). In addition, hepatocyte-conditioned media exhibit potent effects on survival and neurite outgrowth, nearly identical to those of the co-cultured hepatocytes. These findings indicate that hepatocytes secrete a factor that enhances not only neurite regeneration but also neuronal survival. We attempted to purify the hepatocyte-secreted activity using a combination of ultrafiltration, ion exchange chromatography, gel filtration, reverse-phase chromatography, and SDS-PAGE. In extraction experiments, the activity was eluted from an SDS-PAGE gel slice corresponding to a 14-kD protein band. We purified the active ingredient from approximately 1,000 L of culture supernatants of hepatocytes, but the resulting amount of the protein was insufficient for identification of the amino acid sequence (Horie et al., unpublished data).

CONCLUSION

Dissociated cell culture and explant culture systems of adult animal DRG neurons have been utilized as valuable tools for studies on axonal degeneration and regeneration, but the findings from these systems need to be confirmed by *in vivo* experiments. We hope that the review in this chapter will help the researchers in the field of cellular neuroscience to understand the merits and demerits of these culture systems and to make the most of this knowledge.

ACKNOWLEDGMENTS

Our work presented in this chapter was supported by Grants-in-aid for Scientific Research from the Ministry of Education, Science, Technology, Sports, and Culture of Japan (grant numbers 22500324 and 25430056) and was partly performed within the framework of the Cooperative Research Project Program of the Medical Institute of Bioregulation, Kyushu University. We thank Drs. Shuji Inoue, Kazuhiko Watabe, Hitoshi Kawano, and Richard L. Proia for helpful suggestions; Emiko Kawakami, Shizuka Takaku, Hiroko Yanagisawa, Kentaro Endo, and the late Kyoko Ajiki for technical assistance; and Enago (www.enago.jp) for the English language review.

REFERENCES

Averill, S., Davis, D.R., Shortland, P.J., Priestley, J.V. & Hunt, S.P. (2002). Dynamic pattern of reg-2 expression in rat sensory neurons after peripheral nerve injury. *J Neurosci.* 22, 7493-7501.

Averill, S., Inglis, J.J., King, V.R., Thompson, S.W., Cafferty, W.B., Shortland, P.J., Hunt, S.P., Kidd, B.L. & Priestley, J.V. (2008). Reg-2 expression in dorsal root ganglion neurons after adjuvant-induced monoarthritis. *Neuroscience,* 155, 1227-1236.

Cafferty, W.B., McGee, A.W. & Strittmatter, S.M. (2008) Axonal growth therapeutics: regeneration or sprouting or plasticity? *Trends Neurosci.,* 31, 215-220.

Camby, I., Le Mercier, M., Lefranc, F. & Kiss, R. (2006). Galectin-1: a small protein with major functions. *Glycobiology,* 16, 137R-157R.

Campbell, J.E. & Drucker, D.J. (2013). Pharmacology, physiology, and mechanisms of incretin hormone action. *Cell Metab.,* 17, 819-837.

Chowdhury, S.K., Smith, D.R. & Fernyhough, P. (2013). The role of aberrant mitochondrial bioenergetics in diabetic neuropathy. *Neurobiol. Dis.,* 51, 56-65.

Cohen, P.L. & Eisenberg, R.A. (1991). Lpr and gld: single gene models of systemic autoimmunity and lymphoproliferative disease. *Annu. Rev. Immunol.,* 9, 243-269.

Cooper, D.N. & Barondes, S.H. (1990). Evidence for export of a muscle lectin from cytosol to extracellular matrix and for a novel secretory mechanism. *J. Cell Biol.,* 110, 1681-1691.

Curtis, R., Adryan, K.M., Zhu, Y., Harkness, P.J., Lindsay, R.M. & DiStefano, P.S. (1993). Retrograde axonal transport of ciliary neurotrophic factor is increased by peripheral nerve injury. *Nature,* 365, 253-255.

Davis, S., Aldrich, T.H., Stahl, N., Pan, L., Taga, T., Kishimoto, T., Ip, N.Y. & Yancopoulos, G.D. (1993). LIFRβ and gp130 as heterodimerizing signal transducers of the tripartide CNTF receptor. *Science* 260, 1808-1810.

Echigo, Y., Sugiki, H., Koizumi, Y., Hikitsuchi, S. & Inoue, H. (2010). Activation of RAW264.7 macrophages by oxidized galectin-1. *Immunol. Lett.,* 131, 19-23.

Fang, M., Wang, J., Huang, J.Y., Ling, S.C., Rudd, J.A., Hu, Z.Y., Yew, D.T. & Han, S. (2011). The neuroprotective effects of Reg-2 following spinal cord transection injury. *Anat. Rec.,* 294, 24-45.

Ferguson, T.A. & Muir, D. (2000). MMP-2 and MMP-9 increase the neurite-promoting potential of Schwann cell basal laminae and are upregulated in degenerated nerve. *Mol. Cell Neurosci.,* 16, 157-167.

Goldenberg, S.S. & De Boni, U. (1983). Pure population of viable neurons from rabbit dorsal root ganglia, using gradients of Percoll. *J. Neurobiol.,* 14, 195-206.

Halvorsen, S.W. & Kaur, N. (2006). CNTF and related neurokines. In: Lajtha, A. (ed.) Handbook of neurochemistry and molecular neurobiology, 3rd ed. Lim, R. (volume ed.) Neuroactive proteins and peptides, New York; *Springer, Science+Business Media LLC,* pp. 43-68.

Harkavyi, A. & Whitton, P.S. (2010). Glucagon-like peptide 1 receptor stimulation as a means of neuroprotection. *Br. J. Pharmacol.,* 159, 495-501.

Hikawa, N., Kiuchi, Y., Maruyama, T. & Takenaka, T. (1997). Delayed neurite regeneration and its improvement by nerve growth factor (NGF) in dorsal root ganglia from MRL-lpr/lpr mice in vitro. *J. Neurol. Sci.,* 149, 13-17.

Himeno, T., Kamiya, H., Naruse, K., Harada, N., Ozaki, N., Seino, Y., Shibata, T., Kondo, M., Kato, J., Okawa, T., Fukami, A., Hamada, Y., Inagaki, N., Seino, Y., Drucker, D.J., Oiso, Y. & Nakamura, J. (2011).

Beneficial effects of exendin-4 on experimental polyneuropathy in diabetic mice. *Diabetes,* 60, 2397-2406.

Horie, H., Kawasaki, Y. & Takenaka, T. (1986). Lateral diffusion of membrane lipids changes with aging in mouse dorsal root ganglion neurons. *Brain Res.,* 377, 246-250.

Horie, H., Ikuta, S., Takenaka, T. & Ito, S. (1989). Adaptation of cultured mammalian neurons to a hypotonic environment with age-related response. *Brain Res.,* 477, 233-240.

Horie, H., Ikuta, S. & Takenaka, T. (1990). Membrane elasticity of mouse dorsal root ganglion neurons decreases with aging. *FEBS Lett.,* 269, 23-25.

Horie, H., Bando, Y., Chi, H. & Takenaka, T. (1991a). NGF enhances neurite regeneration from nerve-transected terminals of young adult and aged mouse dorsal root ganglia in vitro. *Neurosci. Lett.,* 121, 125-128.

Horie, H., Fukuda, N. & Bando, Y. (1991b). Hepatocytes enhance neurite regeneration and survival from transected nerve terminals. *Neuroreport,* 2, 521-524.

Horie, H., Sango, K., Takano, M. & Takenaka, T. (1993). Response of aged neurons to super-hypotonic environment. *Jpn. J. Physiol.,* 43, S193-S196.

Horie, H., Inagaki, Y., Sohma, Y., Nozawa, R., Okawa, K., Hasegawa, M., Muramatsu, N., Kawano, H., Horie, M., Koyama, H., Sakai, I., Takeshita, K., Kowada, Y., Takano, M. & Kadoya, T. (1999). Galectin-1 regulates initial axonal growth in peripheral nerves after axotomy. *J. Neurosci.,* 19, 9964-9974.

Horie, H. & Kadoya, T. (2000). Identification of oxidized galectin-1 as an initial repair regulatory factor after axotomy in peripheral nerves. *Neurosci. Res.,* 38, 131-137.

Horie, H., Kadoya, T., Hikawa, N., Sango, K., Inoue, H., Takeshita, K., Asawa, R., Hiroi, T., Sato, M., Yoshioka, T. & Ishikawa, Y. (2004). Oxidized galectin-1 stimulates macrophages to promote axonal regeneration in peripheral nerves after axotomy. *J. Neurosci.,* 24, 1873-1880.

Kan, M., Guo, G., Singh, B., Singh, V. & Zochodne, D.W. (2012). Glucagon-like peptide 1, insulin, sensory neurons, and diabetic neuropathy. *J. Neuropathol. Exp. Neurol.,* 71, 494-510.

Kleitman, N., Wood, P.M. & Bunge, R.P. (1998). Tissue culture methods for the study of myelination. In: Banker, G. & Goslin, K. (ed.), *Culturing nerve cells,* 2nd ed. Cambridge: MITP. pp. 545-594.

Kuffler, D.P., Sosa, I.J. & Reyes, O. (2009) Schwann cell chondroitin sulfate proteoglycan inhibits dorsal root ganglion neuron neurite outgrowth and substrate specificity via a soma and not a growth cone mechanism. *J. Neurosci. Res.,* 87, 2863-2871.

Li, Y., Perry, T., Kindy, M.S., Harvey, B.K., Tweedie, D., Holloway, H.W., Powers, K., Shen, H., Egan, J.M., Sambamurti, K., Brossi, A., Lahiri, D.K., Mattson, M.P., Hoffer, B.J., Wang, Y. & Greig, N.H. (2009). GLP-1 receptor stimulation preserves primary cortical and dopaminergic neurons in cellular and rodent models of stroke and Parkinsonism. *Proc. Natl. Acad. Sci. USA,* 106, 1285-1290.

Lindsay, R.M. (1988). Nerve growth factors (NGF, BDNF) enhance axonal regeneration but are not required for survival of adult sensory neurons. *J. Neurosci.,* 8, 2394-2405.

Liu, W.J., Jin, H.Y., Lee, K.A., Xie, S.H., Baek, H.S. & Park, T.S. (2011). Neuroprotective effect of the glucagon-like peptide-1 receptor agonist, synthetic exendin-4, in streptozotocin-induced diabetic rats. *Br. J. Pharmacol.,* 164, 1410-1420.

Manfridi, A., Forloni, G.L., Arrigoni-Martelli, E. & Mancia, M. (1992) Culture of dorsal root ganglion neurons from aged rats: effects of acetyl-L-carnitine and NGF. *Int. J. Dev. Neurosci.,* 10, 321-329.

Mason, M.R., Tannemaat, M.R., Malessy, M.J. & Verhaagen, J. (2011). Gene therapy for the peripheral nervous system: a strategy to repair the injured nerve? *Curr. Gene Therapy,* 11, 75-89.

McClean, P.L., Parthsarathy, V., Faivre, E. & Hölscher, C. (2011). The diabetes drug liraglutide prevents degenerative processes in a mouse model of Alzheimer's disease. *J Neurosci.,* 31, 6587-6594.

Moller, K., Reimer, M., Hannibal, J., Fahrenkrug, J., Sundler, F. & Kanje, M. (1997). Pituitary adenylate cyclase-activating peptide (PACAP) and PACAP type 1 receptor expression in regenerating adult mouse and rat superior cervical ganglia in vitro. *Brain Res.,* 775, 156-165.

Molliver, D.C., Wright, D.E., Leitner, M.L., Parsadanian, A.S., Doster, K., Wen, D., Yan, Q. & Snider, W.D. (1997). IB4-binding DRG neurons switch from NGF to GDNF dependence in early postnatal life. *Neuron,* 19, 849-861.

Nishimune, H., Vasseur, S., Wiese, S., Birling, M.C., Holtmann, B., Sendtner, M., Iovanna, J.L. & Henderson, C.E. (2000). Reg-2 is a motoneuron neurotrophic factor and a signalling intermediate in the CNTF survival pathway. *Nat. Cell Biol.,* 2, 906-914.

Ohsawa, M., Kotani, M., Tajima, Y., Tsuji, D., Ishibashi, Y., Kuroki, A., Itoh, K., Watabe, K., Sango, K., Yamanaka, Y. & Sakuraba, H. (2005). Establishment of immortalized Schwann cells from a Sandhoff mouse and corrective effect of recombinant human b-hexosaminidase A on the accumulated GM2 ganglioside. *J. Human Genet.,* 50, 460-467.

Päiväläinen, S., Nissinen, M., Honkanen, H., Lahti, O., Kangas, S.M., Peltonen, J., Peltonen, S. & Heape, A.M. (2008). Myelination in mouse dorsal root ganglion/Schwann cell cocultures. *Mol. Cell. Neurosci.,* 37, 568-578.

Perry, T., Holloway, H.W., Weerasuriya, A., Mouton, P.R., Duffy, K., Mattison, J.A. & Greig, N,H. (2007). Evidence of GLP-1-mediated neuroprotection in an animal model of pyridoxine-induced peripheral sensory neuropathy. *Exp. Neurol.,* 203, 293-301.

Petersen, M. (1999). Adult rat spinal sensory ganglia, In: L.W. Haynes (Ed), The neuron in tissue culture (pp. 393-398). *Chichester: John Wiley & Sons Ltd.*

Phaneuf, D., Wakamatsu, N., Huang, J.Q., Borowski, A., Peterson, A.C., Fortunato, S.R., Ritter, G., Igdoura, S.A., Morales, C.R., Benoit, G., Akerman, B.R., Leclerc, D., Hanai, N., Marth, J.D., Trasler, J.M. & Gravel, R.A. (1996). Dramatically different phenotypes in mouse models of human Tay-Sachs and Sandhoff diseases. *Hum. Mol. Genet.,* 5, 1-14.

Plachta, N., Annaheim, C., Bissière, S., Lin, S., Rüegg, M., Hoving, S., Müller, D., Poirier, F., Bibel, M. & Barde, Y.A. (2007). Identification of a lectin causing the degeneration of neuronal processes using engineered embryonic stem cells. *Nat. Neurosci.,* 10, 712-719.

Regan, L.J., Dodd, J., Barondes, S.H. & Jessell, T.M. (1986). Selective expression of endogenous lactose-binding lectins and lactoseries glycoconjugates in subsets of rat sensory neurons. *Proc. Natl. Acad. Sci. USA,* 83, 2248-2252.

Saito, H., Sango, K., Horie, H., Takeshita, K., Ikeda, H., Ishigatsubo, Y. & Ishikawa, Y. (2002). Trachea enhances neurite regeneration from adult rat nodose ganglia *in vitro. Life Sci.,* 70, 1935-1946.

Sango, K., Horie, H., Inoue, S., Takamura, Y. & Takenaka, T. (1993). Age-related changes of DRG neuronal attachment to extracellular matrix proteins in vitro. *NeuroReport,* 4, 663-666.

Sango, K., Yamanaka, S., Hoffmann, A., Okuda, Y., Grinberg, A., Westphal, H., McDonald, M.P., Crawley, J.N., Sandhoff, K., Suzuki, K. & Proia, R.L. (1995). Mouse models of Tay-Sachs and Sandhoff diseases differ in neurologic phenotype and ganglioside metabolism. *Nat. Genet.,* 11, 170-176.

Sango, K., Horie, H. & Inoue, S. (1997). Biophysical and biochemical features of diabetic neurons in culture: what have we learned about diabetic neuropathy? *J. Periph. Nerv. Syst.,* 2, 203-211.

Sango, K., Horie, H., Saito, H., Ajiki, K., Tokashiki, A., Takeshita, K., Ishigatsubo, Y., Kawano, H. & Ishikawa, Y. (2002a). Diabetes is not a potent inducer of neuronal cell death in mouse sensory ganglia, but it enhances neurite regeneration in vitro. *Life Sci.,* 71, 2351-2368.

Sango, K., Yamanaka, S., Ajiki, K., Tokashiki, A. & Watabe, K. (2002b). Lysosomal storage results in impaired survival but normal neurite outgrowth in dorsal root ganglion neurons from a mouse model of Sandhoff disease. *Neuropathol. Appl. Neurobiol.,* 28, 23-34.

Sango, K., Oohira, A., Ajiki, K., Tokashiki, A., Horie, M. & Kawano, H. (2003). Phosphacan and neurocan are repulsive substrata for adhesion and neurite extension of adult rat dorsal root ganglion neurons *in vitro*. *Exp. Neurol.,* 182, 1-11.

Sango, K., Tokashiki, A., Ajiki, K., Horie, M., Kawano, H., Watabe, K., Horie, H. & Kadoya, T. (2004). Synthesis, localization and externalization of galectin-1 in mature dorsal root ganglion neurons and Schwann cells. *Eur. J. Neurosci.,* 19, 55-64.

Sango, K., Saito, H., Takano, M., Tokashiki, A., Inoue, S. & Horie, H. (2006). Cultured adult animal neurons and Schwann cells give us new insights into diabetic neuropathy. *Curr. Diabetes Rev.,* 2, 169-183.

Sango, K. (2007). Chondroitin sulfate proteoglycan in the peripheral nervous system after injury. In: *Neural proteoglycans, Maeda, N. (ed.), Kerala; Research Signpost,* pp. 229-238.

Sango, K., Yanagisawa, H. & Takaku, S. (2007). Expression and histochemical localization of ciliary neurotrophic factor in cultured adult rat dorsal root ganglion neurons. *Histochem. Cell Biol.,* 128, 35-43.

Sango, K., Yanagisawa, H., Komuta, Y., Si, Y. & Kawano, H. (2008). Neuroprotective properties of ciliary neurotrophic factor for cultured adult rat dorsal root ganglion neurons. *Histochem. Cell Biol.,* 130, 669-679.

Sango, K., Yanagisawa, H., Kawakami, E., Takaku, S., Ajiki, K., Watabe, K. (2011). Spontaneously immortalized Schwann cells from adult Fischer rat as a valuable tool for exploring neuron-Schwann cell interactions. *J. Neurosci. Res.,* 89, 898-908.

Sango, K., Yanagisawa, H., Watabe, K., Horie, H. & Kadoya, T. (2012). Chapter 3: Galectin-1 as a multifunctional molecule in the peripheral nervous system after injury. In: Rayegani, S.M. (ed.) *Basic Principles of Peripheral Nerve Disorders. Rijeka; InTech doo,* pp 31-46. [http://www.intechopen.com/books/basic-principles-of-peripheral-nerve-disorders/galectin-1-as-a-multifunctional-molecule-in-the-peripheral-nervous-system-after-injury]

Sasaki, T., Hirabayashi, J., Manya, H., Kasai, K. & Endo, T. (2004). Galectin-1 induces astrocyte differentiation, which leads to production of brain-derived neurotrophic factor. *Glycobiology,* 14, 357-363.

Scott, B.S. (1977). Adult mouse dorsal root ganglia neurons in cell culture. *J. Neurobiol.,* 8, 417-427.

Sendtner, M., Carroll, P., Holtmann, B., Hughes, R.A. & Thoenen. H. (1994). Ciliary neurotrophic factor. *J. Neurobiol.,* 25, 1436-1453.

Shuto, T., Horie, H., Hikawa, N., Sango, K., Tokashiki, A., Murata, H., Yamamoto, I. & Ishikawa, Y. (2001). IL-6 up-regulates CNTF mRNA expression and enhances neurite regeneration. *NeuroReport,* 12, 1081-1085.

Starossom, S.C., Mascanfroni, I.D., Imitola, J., Cao, L., Raddassi, K., Hernandez, S.F., Bassil, R., Croci, D.O., Cerliani, J.P., Delacour, D., Wang, Y., Elyaman, W., Khoury, S.J. & Rabinovich, G.A. (2012). Galectin-1 deactivates classically activated microglia and protects from inflammation-induced neurodegeneration. *Immunity,* 37, 249-263.

Taga, T. & Kishimoto, T. (1997). GP130 and the interleukin-6 family of cytokines. *Annu. Rev. Immunol.,* 15, 797-819.

Takaku, S., Yanagisawa, H., Watabe, K., Horie, H., Kadoya, T., Sakumi K., Nakabeppu, Y., Poirier, F. & Sango, K. (2013). GDNF promotes neurite outgrowth and upregulates galectin-1 through the RET/PI3K signaling in cultured adult rat dorsal root ganglion neurons. *Neurochem. Int.,* 62, 330-339.

Terenghi, G. (1999). Peripheral nerve regeneration and neurotrophic factors. *J. Anat.,* 194, 1-14.

Welch, M. & Foster, K. (1999). Embryonic rat spinal sensory ganglia, In: L.W. Haynes (Ed.), The neuron in tissue culture. Chichester; *John Wiley & Sons Ltd.,* pp. 389-393.

Xiao, J., Wong, A.W., Willingham, M.M., Kaasinen, S.K., Hendry, I.A., Howitt, J., Putz, U., Barrett, G.L., Kilpatrick, T.J. & Murray, S.S. (2009). BDNF exerts contrasting effects on peripheral myelination of NGF-dependent and BDNF-dependent DRG neurons. *J. Neurosci.,* 29, 4016-4022.

Yasuda, H., Terada, M., Maeda, K., Kogawa, S., Sanada, M., Haneda, M., Kashiwagi, A. & Kikkawa, R. (2003). Diabetic neuropathy and nerve regeneration. *Prog. Neurobiol.,* 69, 229-285.

Zigmond, R.E. (2011). gp130 cytokines are positive signals triggering changes in gene expression and axon outgrowth in peripheral neurons following injury. *Front. Mol. Neurosci.,* 4, 62.

Zochodne, D. (2008). Neurobiology of Peripheral Nerve Regeneration. Cambridge; *Cambridge University Press.*

Zuo, J., Hernandez, Y.J. & Muir, D. (1998). Chondroitin sulfate proteoglycan with neurite-inhibiting activity is up-regulated following peripheral nerve injury. *J. Neurobiol.,* 34, 41-54.

INDEX

B

C

D

E

F

G

H

O

P

R

S

T

U

V

W

Y